RAWLICIOUS
SUPERFOODS

WITH 100+ RECIPES FOR A HEALTHY LIFESTYLE

RAWLICIOUS
SUPERFOODS

WITH 100+ RECIPES FOR A HEALTHY LIFESTYLE

PETER AND BERYN DANIEL

ILLUSTRATIONS BY ALEXIS ARONSON
FOREWORD BY DAVID WOLFE

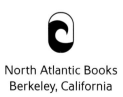

North Atlantic Books
Berkeley, California

Published by
North Atlantic Books
P.O. Box 12327
Berkeley, California 94712

Cover illustration by Alexis Aronson
Cover design by Jasmine Hromjak
Illustrations by Alexis Aronson, alexisaronson.com

Cover photo by Allan M. Photography
Interior design by Marissa Cuenoud and Jasmine Hromjak
All photographs by Peter Daniel unless otherwise noted

Printed in the United States of America

Rawlicious Superfoods: With 100+ Recipes for a Healthy Lifestyle is sponsored and published by the Society for the Study of Native Arts and Sciences (dba North Atlantic Books), an educational nonprofit based in Berkeley, California, that collaborates with partners to develop cross-cultural perspectives, nurture holistic views of art, science, the humanities, and healing, and seed personal and global transformation by publishing work on the relationship of body, spirit, and nature.

North Atlantic Books' publications are available through most bookstores. For further information, visit our website at www.northatlanticbooks.com or call 800-733-3000.

Library of Congress Cataloging-in-Publication Data

Daniel, Peter, 1980-
  Rawlicious superfoods : with 100+ recipes for a healthy lifestyle / Peter and Beryn Daniel ; illustrated by Alexis Aronson.
       pages cm
  Summary: "Cookbook revealing the healing power of superfoods from around the world. Includes photos and illustrations"— Provided by publisher.
  ISBN 978-1-58394-922-1 (pbk.) — ISBN 978-1-58394-923-8 (ebook)
  1. Functional foods. 2. Natural foods. 3. Cooking (Natural foods) I. Daniel, Beryn, 1979- II. Aronson, Alexis. III. Title.
  QP144.F85D36 2015
  613.2--dc23
                     2014024579

1 2 3 4 5 6 7 8 9 VERSA 20 19 18 17 16 15

FOR KATARA—SPIRIT STAR

MAY YOUR WORLD BE FILLED WITH EVER MORE

LOVE AND MAGIC.

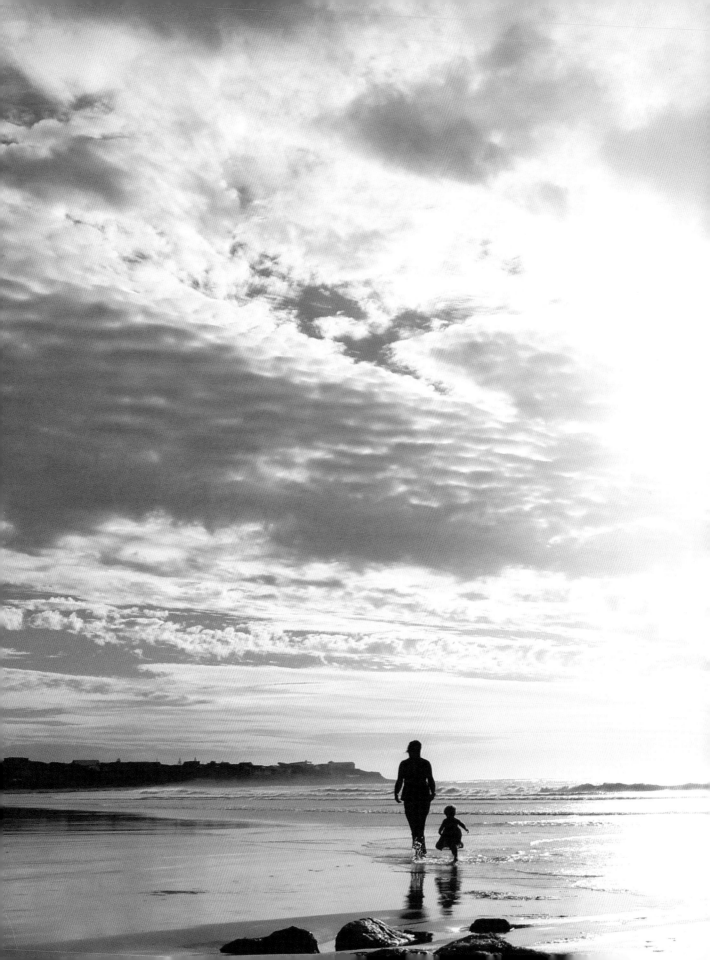

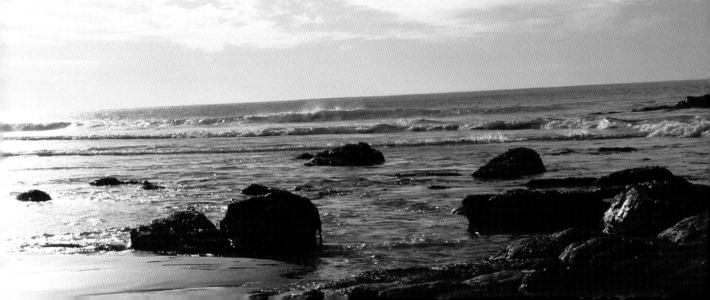

SUPERFOOD MAGIC

Magic to some, common sense to others
A chance to journey and see what's discovered

The earth gifts us form and the nourishment to travel
down the path of discovery of our awesome potential

As bridges between heaven and earth we can be
integrating form with spirit we'll see

The earth's rising power reaches up through darkness
Raw, refining, searching for fulfillment in the vastness

Where the sun beams in glory, transmuting all in time
to ignite the light within us, radiating the eternal divine

Peter Daniel

ACKNOWLEDGMENTS

As raw food chefs, Peter and I could have written a simple recipe book on how to use superfoods. Instead, what you find now within your hands is a work of art. This could not have been possible without the magical input and combined energies of three highly talented and professional artists.

Alexis, it takes power, sight, and wizardry to channel such phenomenal images into form. Each illustration is a masterpiece. The supporting mandalas and doodles are indeed a body of work to behold! Thank you for holding the vision throughout the twelve months it's taken to birth this book, even when Peter and I were unable to focus on it. And just when we thought we were nearing the end, you amazed us with your poetry—a literary sparkle in the eye of each superfood.

Marissa, thank you for bringing it all together with design integrity. Between Peter, Lex, and me, we put illustrations, poetry, technical information, recipes, photographs, doodles, and fun facts into your cauldron; with a wave of your magic wand out came a cohesive, magnificent book. To weave together such apparently contrasting visual elements is akin to defeating the dragon, making you the behind-the-scenes heroine of the day!

Luke, there are not many professional photographers who will work around the schedule of a sixteen-month-old until the task is done! Luckily for us, we have one in the family who is not only patient but incredibly passionate and talented as well. Thanks for taking thousands of photographs in pursuit of getting that perfect shot!

To the team at North Atlantic Books, thank you for your continuous support, hours of effort, and for helping the superfoods message go global!

THANKS

From Peter and Beryn Daniel:
To Katara, our spirit star, for bringing light, love, and inspiration wherever you go!

To our parents for being those extra pairs of hands that helped us to contain and entertain her light whilst we were elbow-deep in ingredients. At last, as parents ourselves, we can appreciate the depth of love and support you share with us daily and forever.

To everyone at Soaring Free Superfoods for placing wings on each package of superfoods and sending it out into the world with love. Your commitment of time, energy, and attention to the daily details has given us the freedom to reach into the creative unknown and bring back this book.

To Avo, for writing the best-ever foreword for this book, and for trailblazing the path along which the superfoods have been able to do their work. Thank you for your inspiration and the dedication to the work that you do.

To our brothers Werner and Callan, thank you for bringing your energy, enthusiasm, love, and lightness to our lives and the superfood message every day.

To Kerry, Peter, and Joshua, thank you for your consistent reflecting and mirroring, for full circles and friendship. Josh, thanks for being my chocolate buddy in the kitchen.

To Barbara, Natalie, Noel, Matt, Lexi, and Werner, thank you for your sensational recipe contributions to this book, and for living and breathing the magic of superfoods along with us.

To our superfood suppliers, thank you for planting, growing, harvesting, and processing the best superfoods in the world, and then sending them to the farthest tip of Africa! Thanks for your attention to detail and for taking loving care of our planet in your efforts to deliver to us from her bounty.

A big thank you goes out to all readers and supporters of our first book, *Rawlicious*. To our customers and event participants, thanks for listening to our zany ideas about food and health and for being brave enough to try them out and radiate the benefits to others. Together we are the difference that makes the difference!

And then, of course, there are the superfoods themselves, all living, magical beings, plants that draw nutrients up from deep in our precious earth and transform radiant sunshine into edible life. We feel truly grateful and blessed to be ambassadors and tools through which you silently and powerfully weave magic and health into the fabric of our cells.

From Alexis Aronson:
Infinite and resounding thanks to my family: Mom, Dad, Granny, Bobby, Spannie, Jamie, and Claire. No amount of thanking I do in words can match the depth of your giving and the force of your love.

Jessie and Shans, fine featherless friends of my heart, my playmates and traveling companions, my inspiration in things arty, my besties on forest paths and city streets, thank you for seeing it all and loving me enough to still want more!

Nedyah, for being part of this journey (from seed to sprout to blossoming and fruition) and for all that we have shared.

Bcryn and Peter, as friends, as family, and as co-creators, for spurring this vision into being, for your belief and acceptance, humility and grace, and for pursuing the gold in yourselves in a way that inspires and supports others in the same ascending spiral. And, of course, thanks for the Bundle!

Marissa, for fine music taste, good laughs, and for being the one through whom it all comes together (no small feat, that).

Murray, who let himself be the faeries' emissary on the spur of the moment and helped me get my pencils. The universe works!

Brian Froud, for listening to the creatures of the imagination and the otherworld, and for one sage and rosy-nosed green man who found his way into the drawings.

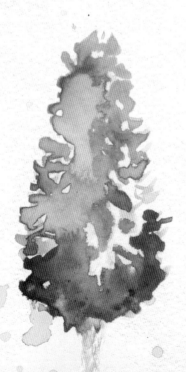

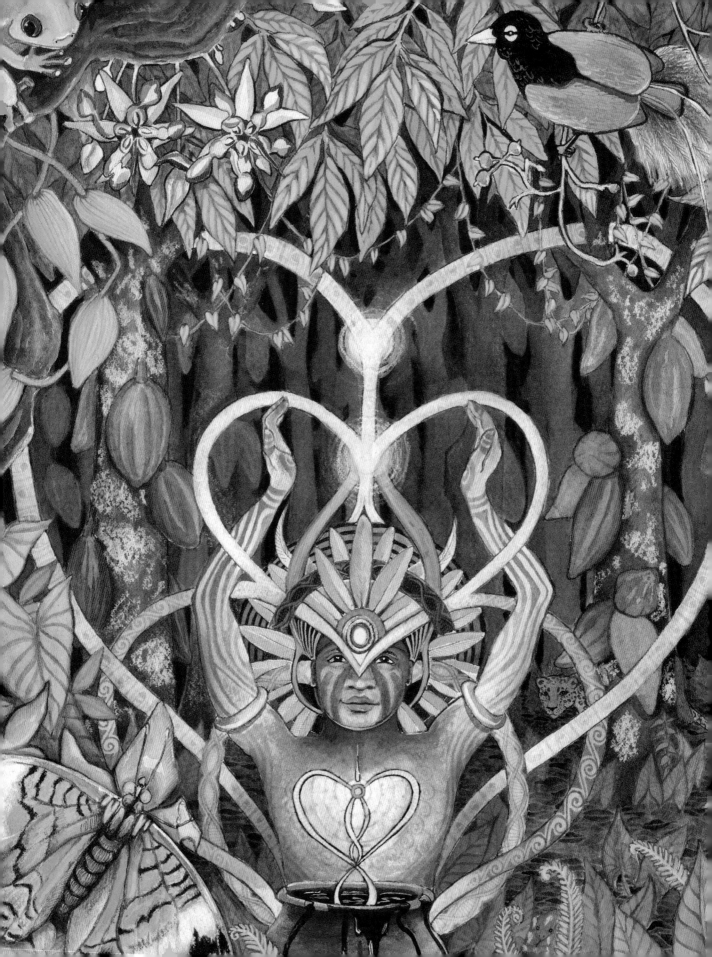

TABLE OF CONTENTS

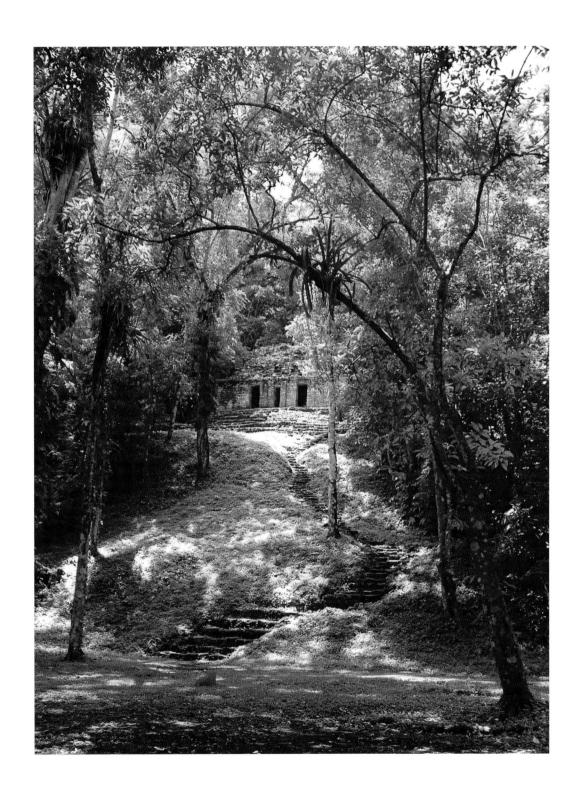

FOREWORD

Superfoods are arriving just in time. Today's world is radically different from the world we knew before the Internet, let alone the world that existed before the television set or the automobile. And because of our changing world and environment, our food choices must change in order to meet the demands of our new world.

Each new generation has been handed the task to review, correct, and perfect the path they've been handed by the previous. Inevitably, in our era, a review of all food history has given rise to the discovery of superfoods: a food category designed to nourish (in all ways) those individuals who have been waiting to take their lives to the next level. In humanity's relentless pursuit of perfection, progress is being made.

Superfoods are the greatest foods identified by the greatest civilizations that have existed on earth. For example, the extraordinary unknown histories of American cultures were nourished with chia seeds and chocolate seeds (cacao beans); the presence of these superfoods in our world now represents the contribution of these cultures to the future—which is now.

In these pages, Peter and Beryn test the food solutions at the fringes of our collective awareness with superfoods that directly relate to personal and planetary solutions. They speak to one of our deepest longings in all aspects of our lives: a reconnection to the origin, to the sacred. Superfoods are sacred foods.

As Peter and Beryn relate, each superfood has its repertoire of benefits, interesting compound nutrients, exotic histories, as well as fascinating flavors and recipes. I am, personally, so fascinated by superfoods that I have experimented with growing practically all of them in gardens and orchards. I recommend you do as well.

Peter and Beryn are deeply involved with the subject matter. For them superfoods have been food for the family for years: "Aloe isn't a food; it's a way of life." The recipes in this book are tried and tested. That's why you will appreciate them so much. The delivery of each detail concerning every superfood is intimate and timely.

Perhaps the most practical parts of this book are the superfood recipes. These are so wonderful and powerful, your imagination will activate. These recipes might turn you into a Mayan Technicolor dream queen for a few hours or an Incan messenger in the mists of the Andes, fueled by maca and berries. These are recipes and formulas that seize the day and inspire a momentary bio-chemical enlightenment.

Blended into the crucible of spring waters—or even coconut waters—the blended protein drinks of yesteryear give way to the superfood smoothies and the superfood-superherb delights of today. Opening up to these culinary marvels is opening up to grace. Maybe there is a reason, all over the world, these superfoods seem to emerge as pageantry in the health press. Let them dazzle you with their brilliance.

Enjoy the pure joy and wonder of Peter and Beryn's information and recipes, and have The Best Day Ever!

David "Avocado" Wolfe
October 2013, Ontario, Canada

www.davidwolfe.com
Author of:
Superfoods: The Food and Medicine of the Future
Eating for Beauty
Naked Chocolate
Longevity Now: A Comprehensive Approach to Healthy Hormones, Detoxification, Super Immunity, Reversing Calcification, and Total Rejuvenation

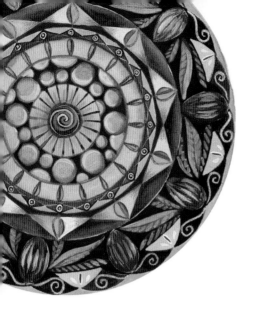

INTRODUCTION

We live in an amazing time. The nutritional opportunities available to us are awesome; we have access to foods that in the recent past were reserved for those few who had the wealth or knowledge to access them from afar, or to the indigenous peoples who have used them for thousands of years. Pioneering research into the field of nutrition, combined with the ancient healing systems of the world, bring us the most prized foods available on earth: foods that are now becoming mainstream news, foods that bring the healing gifts at a time most needed. Chemical agriculture, chemical living, and chemical medicine have failed to live up to their promise of better health through technology; ineffective technology has separated us from our greater body—the earth—and poisoned both to shocking proportions. Most food available today is a pale shadow of the vibrant, nutrient-dense originals eaten by our great-grandparents. It seems crazy, but the older you are the more likely you are to be healthy. Children are being born today with over 250 toxic chemicals in their blood from day one! That's a lot for a small body to cope with. The parents provided the chemicals from their toxic bodies, and combined with widespread nutritional deficiencies it's no wonder disease rates are skyrocketing.

> And we have made of ourselves living cesspools and driven doctors to invent names for our diseases.
>   Plato

How many pills does someone need to take before realizing, "I am not getting the results I expected"? It's time to take the real pill, designed over thousands of years by Mother Nature herself. Recognized by our bodies as friends and helpers, they have been offering themselves as food for thousands of years. Our bodies recognize the gift, revel in the nourishment, and awaken to the memory of an ancient relationship. This ancient relationship has been passed down by traditional healers to this day, but it has been reduced to a secret that is not allowed to be told. Not allowed! The ancient knowledge that food can heal and is therapeutic can't be hidden. The powerful spirits that embody the superfoods laugh in the face of ridiculous legislation intent on dumbing down society to accept that food cannot heal. Western corporate "food" and "medicine" masquerade as the pinnacle of our technological achievement, yet the evidence of monumental failure is all around us. Who does not know someone with an incurable disease?

Most of us do. It's time to go back to tried and tested technologies that have been around for thousands of years. Herbalism: The earth's plants are food *and* medicine. Combine them daily as nourishment and you have what traditional medicine calls "tonic herbalism." Eat the top few superfoods and herbs from these ancient systems daily, and slowly remove the empty, lifeless, nutrient-deficient foods from your diet.

> *Let food be thy medicine and let thy medicine be food.*
>   *Hippocrates*

With this simple process, magic happens—magic that is really just common sense. Once the body becomes clean and nourished, it works!

> *The body heals itself and nutrition provides the resources to accomplish the task.*
>   *Roger Williams, PhD*

The radical health changes we have witnessed in ourselves and people who have embraced this approach motivated us to bring it to life in this book. The energy of these ancient beings has worked through us, becoming what our cells are made of. They express the simple truth that nature has the answers. The farther we stray from nature, the deeper we descend into disease. We invite you to join us on this exciting journey of discovery into a world of lightness and fun, revealing the ancient wisdom that can inspire us to balance and integrity.

> *Vitality and beauty are gifts of nature for those who live according to its laws.*
>   *Leonardo da Vinci*

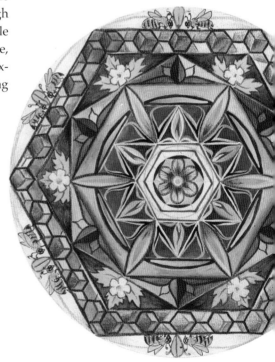

OUR JOURNEY WITH SUPERFOODS

PETER: MY SUPERFOOD STORY

I was first introduced to superfoods while in the UK. We were at a health trade show and one of the exhibitors asked me if I had tried goji berries before. I had not. They were pleasant enough, but there was certainly no big "wow" moment. I did some research that night and was amazed at how powerful goji berries are. This motivated me to eat them regularly, and I believe that because of this I was guided to find the raw food lifestyle years later and eventually teach people about raw foods and superfoods. Interestingly, the Chinese name for goji berries means "school of learning," and it is said that eating them teaches you about herbal medicine.

My most significant memory of superfoods is finding out about raw cacao online. I was searching for a chocolate alternative for Beryn, as she had decided to kick the habit, and I found a website about "raw cacao." The person proclaiming the health benefits of raw cacao was David Wolfe, an international expert in the field of nutrition. I bought some cacao nibs online and never looked back! I met David at a retreat in the UK a few months later and was inspired by his energy to pursue this lifestyle.

Another memory is of my fight with the UK's top superfood. While gardening one day I brushed a plant that caused my hand to break out in itchy stings! That was my first introduction to stinging nettles. I spent hours pulling them out of my garden, thinking "What a nasty plant!" It was only years later that I discovered how profound a superfood it is and that I should have been encouraging its growth!

Since then Beryn and I have had so many magical experiences visiting remote places to see where the superfoods grow—the cacao jungles of Ecuador, the deep Gobi Desert behind the Himalayas in China in search of wild gojis, and the wild African bush for *Aloe ferox* and ancient baobabs.

I have been presenting workshops and seminars on superfoods for years now and continue to be amazed by these profound wonders of nature.

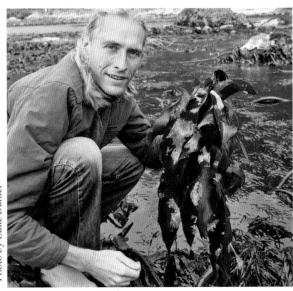

Photo by Luke Daniel

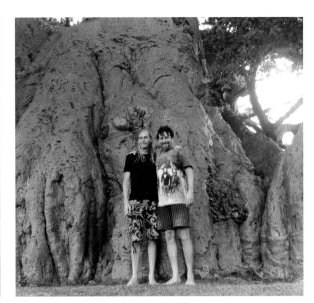

BERYN: MY SUPERFOOD STORY

I grew up in a bakery as a complete chocoholic. In my early twenties, at a health trade fair in London, I met Jason Vale, who was promoting his new book *Chocolate Busters* and revealing the health hazards of consuming mass-marketed chocolate. I decided then and there it was time to quit my bad chocolate habit.

As if by magic, I was presented with the alternative. Peter was shopping online and stumbled across raw cacao nibs, which were only just starting to become available in the UK. He ordered some, and a few days later they were delivered to our door. I snacked on raw cacao nibs and raisins and really enjoyed the deep chocolate flavor, sweetened only by the taste of the raisins. I followed the trail of cacao crumbs and quickly discovered the growing raw food and superfood movements. Goji berries, maca powder, wheatgrass, and cacao quickly became part of my daily routine.

Peter and I attended a raw chefs training course, and the wonder of raw foods and superfoods was unveiled to us. I had the true pleasure of tasting a decadent raw chocolate ganache tart made using raw cacao powder—it changed my life! As soon as I realized I didn't have to give up chocolate, and that eating healthily included (and not excluded) delicious and indulgent taste sensations, I embarked with vigor on this new raw food path. Our lives have been transformed by this magical superfood. We moved home to South Africa and started teaching raw food courses. But how could we share our passion without sharing our newly discovered raw cacao recipes? Raw cacao was unavailable and unheard of, so we started importing it, along with goji berries, which we sold at markets and at our raw food courses. Our Superfoods brand and Superfoods import company have grown out of these humble beginnings, and we now have a wide range of the world's best superfoods available throughout the country so that more people can access the health message of superfoods.

I am happy to say that I am still a chocoholic, but a raw and healthy one!

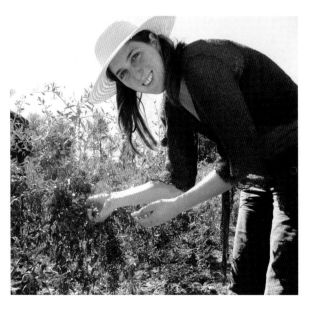

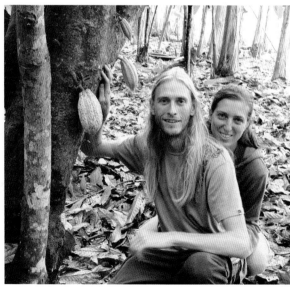

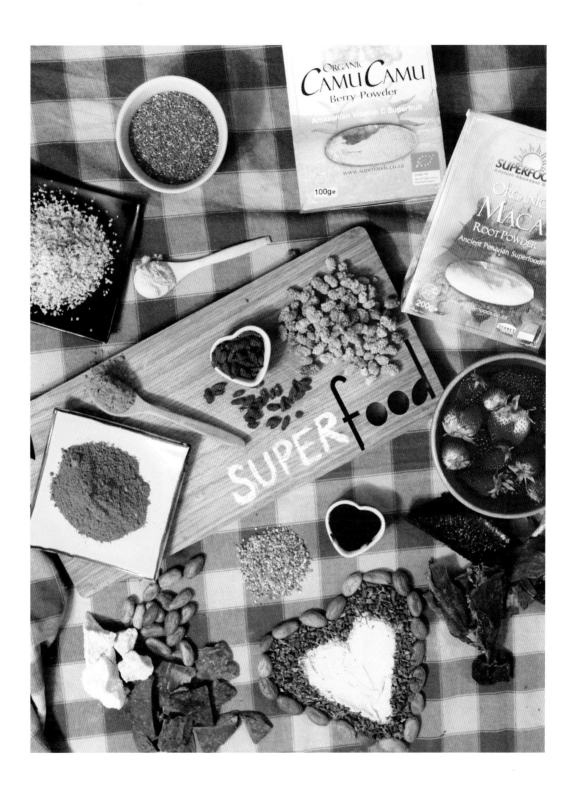

WHAT ARE SUPERFOODS?

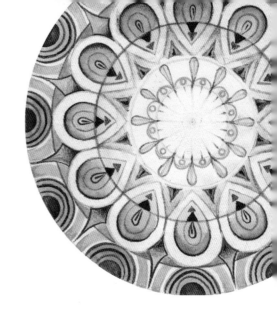

su·per·food | ˈso͞opərˌfo͞od |
noun
a nutrient-rich food considered to be especially beneficial for
  health and well-being.

Superfoods are foods that deliver more: more nutrients, energy, and healing. They are foods that have been revered by ancient cultures around the world for thousands of years, foods that have stood the test of time as healing and nourishing to the human body and been recognized by ancient medicinal systems over generations of experience. Western science is verifying the nutrient density of these foods, and numerous studies are showing the incredible healing ability of their nutrients. These are foods that come from the world's top energetic places: the Amazon rainforest, the top of the Andes Mountains, the foothills of the Himalayas, the wild African plains. Although superfoods are healing in a medicinal way, they are also nourishing. They fill the gap between food and herbal medicine.

> *Superfoods are a major focal point of nutrition because they not*
> *only help nourish the brain, bones, muscles, skin, hair, nails,*
> *heart, lungs, liver, kidneys, reproductive system, pancreas, and*
> *immune system, they also, over the long term, correct imbalances*
> *and help to guide us toward a more natural and aboriginal diet.*
>   *David Wolfe*

There are many foods that have been called superfoods. We have chosen to focus on plant-based superfoods that have a history of traditional use verifying their nourishing ability. These are certainly not the only superfoods out there. Every biome worldwide has its own superfoods that have been used by the indigenous peoples of the area. Find out what they are and use your local heritage!

WHY SUPERFOODS?

Food is no longer food. What we mean is that farming has changed so radically over the past seventy years that what people now eat and accept as food is usually a substance that has very little to no resemblance to the food we have been eating for generations before. The advent of chemical agriculture has meant that soils are depleted of essential trace minerals and soil organisms, resulting in food that looks pretty but is actually severely lacking in nutritional density, especially mineral density. Research has shown that the trace minerals in fruits and vegetables have fallen by up to 80% since 1940. On top of this, the use of toxic biocides continues to rise, exposing people to poisons that the human body has never before been exposed to. On top of all this, big food companies take this low-quality food and further process it into a myriad of highly refined junk foods.

It's no wonder disease rates continue to rise. When the body does not get the nutrients it needs to sustain itself, disease is the result. The food supplement industry has emerged as the supposed answer to the problem of poor food quality. The level of consciousness that caused the problem (chemical farming) cannot solve the problem with the same level of consciousness (chemical food supplements). A large percentage of food supplements are manufactured using cheap ingredients that are very difficult for the body to digest. These chemical supplements also completely ignore the fact that nutrients in food do not function in isolation. We are only just beginning to realize the level of complexity of synergistic actions of the nutrients naturally found together in food. The mechanistic reductionist approach to nutrients misses the point. Nature is a fractal biological system with all parts working in harmony to achieve far more than the sum of those parts.

Chemical supplements also have no DNA and no information. Research is showing that the DNA in food actually transfers information to our own DNA. Lifeless, dead, inorganic nutrient copies will never provide what the body needs. Our bodies have evolved over the millennia to absorb nutrients from food.

One of the most profound ways to improve your health is to change to organic food. Besides the higher level of trace minerals and nutrients, the pesticide content of organic food is 180 times lower. There really is no option if you care about your health. Moving on from there, decades of eating nutrient-deficient foods have left a large deficit in most people's nutrient balances. Something is needed to quickly boost nutrient levels and restore balance. Enter the *superfoods*. They are incredibly nutrient-rich, and are food, so the body can utilize the nutrients.

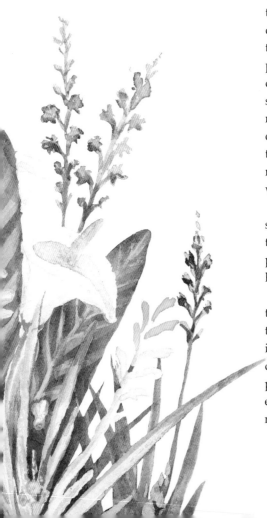

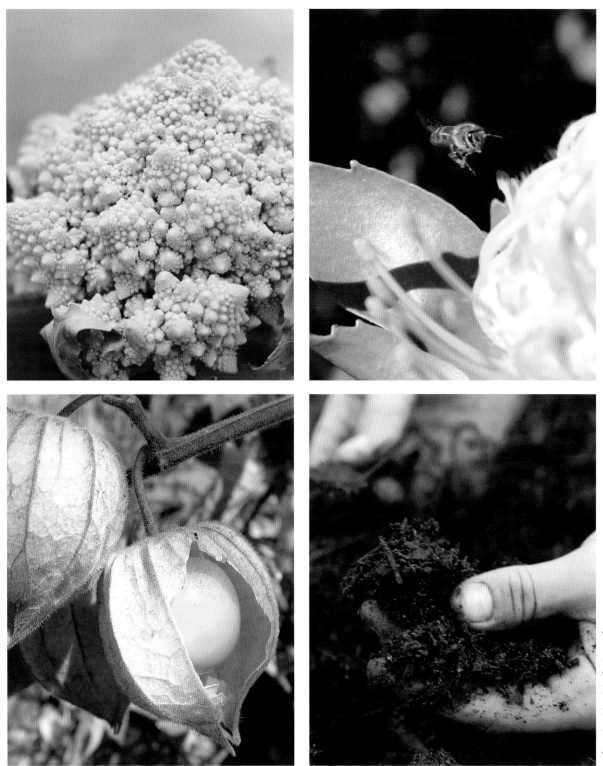

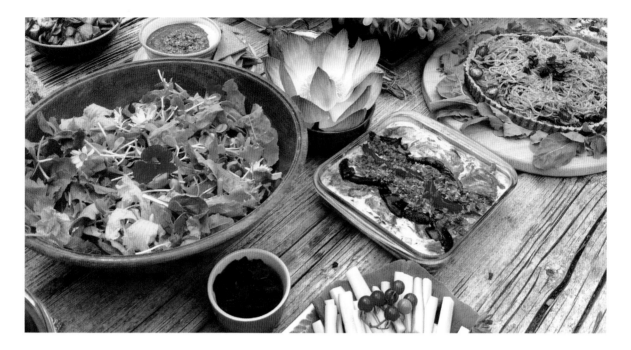

FUNCTIONAL FOOD

Functional food: food that serves more than just the purpose of making you feel full or that you spend some time chewing. Functional food serves the more obvious, yet strangely not so common, purpose of nourishing the body with essential nutrients. In our first book, *Rawlicious*, we describe the raw food lifestyle. The raw food diet is a core component of that lifestyle and is based on a very simple concept. Out of the millions of creatures that walk this earth, we humans are the only ones that cook our food. We are also the only ones that suffer with degenerative diseases en masse. The raw food diet focuses on raw nutrient-dense plants such as fruits, vegetables, nuts, seeds, seaweeds, sprouts, herbs, and superfoods. Emphasis is placed on eating green leafy vegetables by either juicing or blending them. Choosing organic food is almost more important than keeping it raw, as conventional food has so little nutritional value to begin with. Even if you cook organic food, you will likely still be left with far more than what the conventional food started out with.

Many studies show that cooking destroys nutrients. The hotter the food, the more nutrition that is lost. In our talks and seminars we suggest aiming for at least a 50% raw component in the diet, which is easy to do by just adding in a daily fresh juice, smoothie, salad, and a raw snack such as a trail mix or fresh fruits. The rest can be made up of organic vegetables and grains that have been water-cooked by lightly steaming or boiling, or by low-temperature baking. Water-cooking is the least damaging to food. Dry cooking in ovens, toasters, frying pans, and microwaves destroys a large amount of nutrients. Also, toxins such as acrylamide start to form in foods when cooked above 248°F (120°C).

Raw animal foods are sometimes appropriate and needed for some people: foods such as true free-range, organic eggs; raw fermented dairy kefir, especially from Guernsey cows; and the occasional wild-caught raw fish or wild oysters. Extra care must be taken when purchasing animal foods, as they are higher in the food chain and therefore concentrate more environmental toxicity.

This type of foundational diet can super-accelerate a healing process and provide essential nutrient density to stay cleansed and healthy in the short to medium term. For those who want to keep it light and clean for the long term, herbs and superfoods are an essential addition. Our ancestral diet was based on wild food, which is incredibly nutrient dense. Domesticated plant foods may not be able to provide enough nutritional variation for someone to maintain a raw plant-based diet long term. Medicinal herbs and superfoods still have their wild roots present and are incredibly nutrient dense, making up the balance of the equation.

What we also like about superfoods is that, even if you don't want to change your baseline diet, you can just add the superfoods in to still get great benefits. It's also super easy to just add them in—a raw cacao superfood smoothie is simple and quick to make and delicious!

What we have realized is that there are really just three questions to ask about a food to know if it's "good" food:

1. Is the food nutrient dense? Has it been grown organically in nutrient-rich soils and of a cultivar that still has some wild origins left?
2. Is the food clean? Is it free of chemicals such as flavorings, colorants, preservatives, dyes, GMOs, and biocides? Some don't realize that pesticides kill indiscriminately. The only reason people don't die outright from eating pesticides on food is that a human is bigger than an insect and so can handle a higher dose!
3. Is the food undamaged? Having gone to the effort of taking care of the first two questions, zapping food in an oven or microwave and destroying the nutritional value would be a huge waste.

It's really that simple. So next time you are shopping, making a meal, or about to eat a meal, just ask yourself the above three questions. You may be shocked at just how unhealthy most commonly eaten foods are!

WHERE IS THE PROOF?

Western minds are skeptical, and for good reason. There are many snake oil salespeople promising the elixir of youth. What makes the superfoods different is the history of use in traditional medicinal systems. They have been verified by use over thousands of years.

For those who want the numbers, research has been done. However, long-term human studies on specific biomarkers is not only extremely expensive to do, but also very difficult to coordinate and then to link to specific nutrient actions.

We have chosen to keep this book as simple as possible, giving you ideas to look into further. A simple Internet search will bring up thousands of results, and a number of books have also been written on superfoods, listing research studies done. For ease of reference, we will keep an updated list of further reading on our website for those who wish to delve deeper into the whys and hows.

Although each superfood chapter lists specific healing functions generally attributed to that food by historical use or research findings, the superfoods' main action of healing is to nourish the body. This action is often non-specific, meaning all body systems benefit and improve. With this baseline understanding we however list specific actions for each superfood, as they do also vary in nutrient makeup and will therefore have variations in specific actions. The final word on therapeutic benefits will be the results you achieve. If consistent use does not improve your situation, try something else! Not all superfoods will work for all people—we each have unique needs. The consistent feedback we have received over the years from people who use the superfoods is that they have a feeling of greater energy, clarity, and vitality, which are the foundation of health and wellness.

WHAT ABOUT COST?

Over the years of importing superfoods, we have realized a few things about cost. The true cost of producing poor-quality, poison-covered food and depleting soils of life and nutrients with chemicals is enormous. Generations ahead will be flabbergasted at this madness. Real food is more expensive because it is more expensive to produce—due to the use of natural composts and fertilizers, heirloom seeds, and small-scale production methods. It is also far richer in nutrients, making its value much higher than "chem-food."

We love local food and grow many of the superfoods ourselves. Some, however, won't grow in our ecosystem. This is where we don't throw the baby out with the bathwater. The global transportation network has allowed us access to these amazing foods. Food represents only a fraction of the total mass of shipped goods globally, and dried or powdered foods an even smaller fraction of that. If you really want to be more carbon-friendly, buy a locally produced car, appliances, and even clothing. Sea freight is also far less carbon-intensive than air freight. Shipping dried food is also key, as water weight can amount to more than 80% of the original food weight. I recently found that fresh blueberries can be three times more expensive than dried goji berries once you've dehydrated them!

What I love about superfoods is that, although it takes carbon to ship them, they allow us to be more nutritionally balanced, opening our awareness to avoiding environmentally destructive chem-food. They also provide huge amounts of easily digestible protein, reducing the need to consume animal foods, which have been found to be one of the highest contributors to greenhouse gases.

And then there is the cost of quality sourcing. Business moves in two ways: quality and quantity. Trailblazers often take care to source products of the highest quality and integrity, supporting farmers and the earth for the best results for all. Once the word gets out, others jump on the bandwagon with inferior items driven by demand. I have personally tested various superfood brands and found high levels of pesticide residue in so-called organic superfoods. Supporting certified organic brands also supports indigenous farmers to grow certified organic food. Some superfoods, such as heirloom cacao, also preserve forests, as they grow better when planted under the forest canopy.

At the end of the day, it is up to each person to decide if it is worth cutting corners for his or her wallet. We believe that the only option is to feed ourselves foods of the highest quality, nutrient density, and integrity. Remember, when you experience hunger, it is because your body is looking for minerals, amino acids, and other building blocks with which to build your cells, tissues, muscles, etc. When you eat for quality and nutrient density, your body turns off the hunger signals and you feel satiated and satisfied, often for the first time in years! Although enjoying our food is key, we eat to live, not vice versa, and by putting the best-quality fuel into our bodies, we give ourselves the smoothest and most enjoyable life-ride.

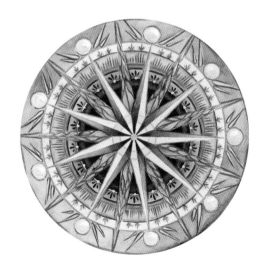

QUALITY IS KEY

- Start reading labels. If you don't understand or cannot pronounce the words on the label, it's best to leave it on the shelf.
- When we refer to fresh ingredients, we mean organic or homegrown wherever possible. Juices should be freshly squeezed.
- The best water to drink is from a natural spring. We collect our own and store it in glass in a cool area of the kitchen, covered with a cloth to keep light out.
- Herbs and spices should be non-irradiated and preferably organic.
- Oils should be extra virgin, cold-pressed, and organic.
- Salt should be Himalayan rock salt or unbleached, non-iodated sea salt.
- Soy-based products such as tamari or miso must be organic and non-GM (genetically modified).
- All dried fruits should be preservative- and sulfur dioxide-free.
- All cacao should be truly raw, having been prepared from raw cacao beans and cold-processed.
- All honey should be raw and unheated.
- With the current controversy around the agave industry, we have decided to use honey, maple syrup, or dates to sweeten dishes.
- Maple syrup should be pure Canadian maple syrup and not maple-flavored syrup.
- When we refer to hot water, we mean parboiled water that has not been heated over 158°F (70°C).
- We avoid all pasteurized foods, as this means they have been cooked.

> *Quality is never an accident. It is always the result of high intention, sincere effort, intelligent direction, and skillful execution; it represents the wise choice of many alternatives.*
> Willa A. Foster

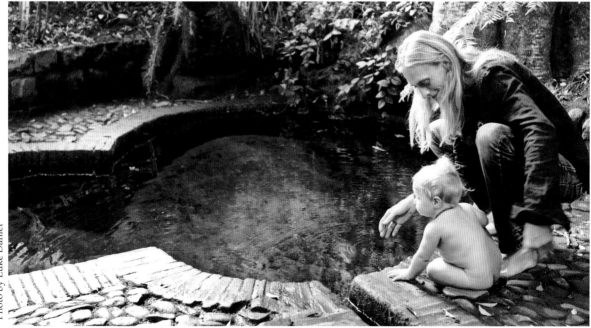

Photo by Luke Daniel

HOW TO USE THIS BOOK

MAGIC INTO BEING

We have been ingesting the nutritional potency of superfoods for years now, and we feel it throughout the cells of our bodies and beings. Since the birth of our daughter Katara (eighteen months at time of writing) we felt the desire to write this superfoods book. As new parents and zany superfoodists, we wanted this book to be extra special and extra fun—something that children could engage with and enjoy too!

We thought of characterizing each superfood as a superhero, and approached our friend and incredibly talented artist, Lexi, to see if she would be interested in the project. Excited, she suggested not superheroes, but illustrations that would capture the magic and essence of each superfood and bring it to life.

When we began to brainstorm, we realized that superfoods are so much more than just superheroes. Yes, they have reappeared at a challenging time and they have "come to save the day," but they represent ancient wisdom, knowledge, and abundance. They represent a connectedness to the earth, the sacred, and the divine. Each magical superfood illustration has a corresponding mandala and has been inspired by hours of discussion around its historical use, medicinal benefits, and mythology. Lexi has poured love, life, and detail into each of these magnificent illustrations. We hope they will delight you and your loved ones as much as they do us.

SIXTEEN SUPERFOODS

We have chosen sixteen superfoods to focus on in this book.

Each superfood section has been designed to weave together all aspects of what makes it a superfood and how to use it. Each illustration page is intended to be a summary of the superfood's essence and its health benefits. The information pages that follow provide details about the ancient revered nature of the superfood as well as the magic of its nutritional aspects and benefits. Peter has researched and refined this information to be easily accessible and digestible.

The recipe sections map out simple, delicious, rawlicious ways of adding the superfood into your daily routine. We have been eating and enjoying these superfoods in so many variations for so many years that the time has finally arrived to write them down in one place!

As herbalists say: compliance is key. You can't get the benefits unless you actually eat them on a regular basis. There is no one-shot wonder pill. The key is to have fun playing with superfoods and discovering which ones work best for you.

Enjoy your journey with superfoods!

MEASUREMENTS

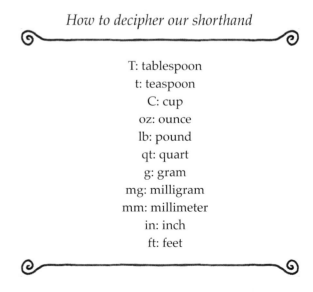

How to decipher our shorthand

T: tablespoon
t: teaspoon
C: cup
oz: ounce
lb: pound
qt: quart
g: gram
mg: milligram
mm: millimeter
in: inch
ft: feet

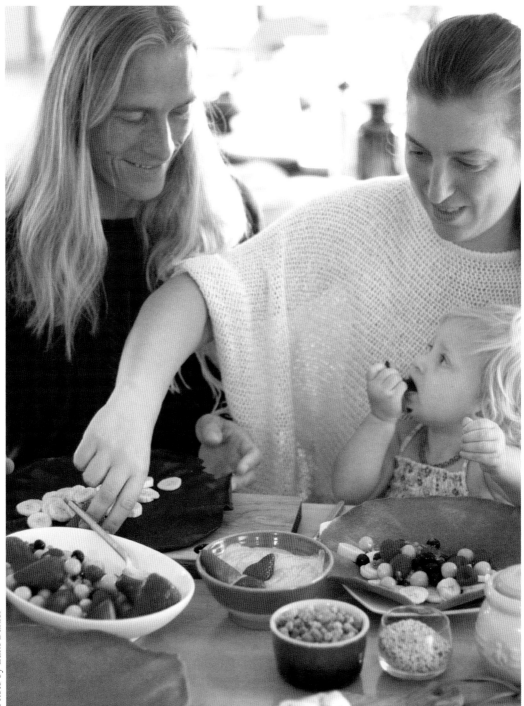

A SUPERFOODIST'S KITCHEN

There are a few things that are good to have when you embark on your superfood adventure. Sharp knives are always a good start, but probably the best and most important piece of equipment to really get tucked into a superfood lifestyle is a blender. The superfood alchemy happens in the blender, where you can synergistically combine the power of a variety of superfoods and superherbs.

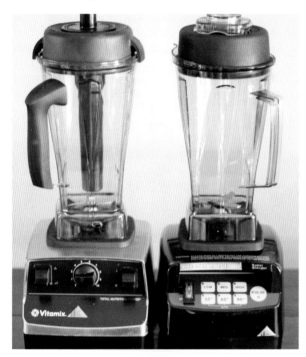

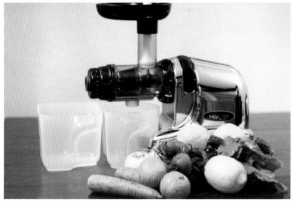

There should be no excuse and no barrier to entry. Start with what you've got! This could be a hand-stick blender or a simple entry-level blender, juicer, or food processor—the key is to start!

When you are ready to gear up, my recommendation would be to invest in a high-speed power blender. You will never look back!

Here is a list of equipment you will find in our kitchen.

BLENDERS

Vitamix

The Rolls Royce of power blenders, enjoyed by blender chefs around the world, is the Vitamix. No other blender I have come across blends as smoothly as a Vitamix.

Hi Blend or Saluté

This machine is able to perform similar functions at a more affordable price.

What distinguishes these blenders from others is that they have a tamper, which enables you to grind the food up against the blades of the jug. By doing so, you can create not only smoothies, but also nut butters, smooth desserts, savory sauces, pestos, soups, chocolate mousse, and so much more.

JUICERS

Oscar juicer

Our machine of choice is a single-auger masticating juicer that slowly grinds the fruit, vegetable, or wheatgrass up against a juicing screen, extracting maximum juice out of even the most fibrous blades of wheatgrass. This machine also comes with a flat grinding plate that can be used for powderizing nuts or creating ice creams out of frozen fruit.

FOOD PROCESSORS

Magimix

A trusty friend in any kitchen, you can do a whole host of things with a food processor, including pulsing, chopping, grating, slicing, and blending. Mostly, it is used in this recipe book for making superfood snack bars, cakes, pestos, crackers, and other sweet and savory delicacies.

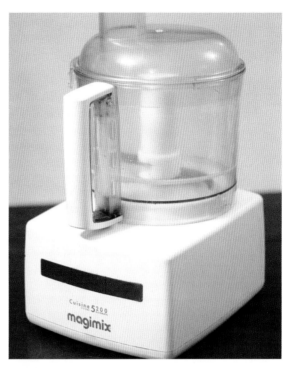

DEHYDRATORS

Excalibur and Ezi-dri

This is a raw foodist's version of an oven. It slowly removes moisture from food at a temperature that can be set below 117°F (47°C), meaning the enzymes and nutrients of the original food remain intact. We have used an Excalibur dehydrator as our dryer in this book and it is our dehydrator of choice. You can remove trays from this box-shaped machine, giving you space and height to dehydrate large dishes. An Ezi-dri Ultra or Snackmaker are equally good dehydrator options. You will need teflex solid sheets. With a dehydrator you can make recipes such as kale chips; hemp bread; hemp burgers; chia, tomato, and onion crackers; macaroons; mesquite banana bread; and so much more!

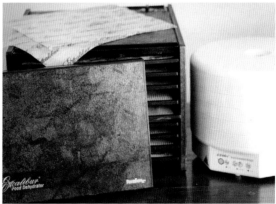

MIRON GLASS

Most powdered superfoods last and store well—in some cases up to two years. The best way to store your superfoods once you get them home to your kitchen is in glass. The absolute best way to store them is in Miron glass. It is the most advanced glass worldwide for storing and energizing foods and liquids. It is a dark purple-violet glass that does not allow light from the visible spectrum to penetrate. Besides just protecting against decomposition, Miron assists in the preservation and stimulation of bioenergy.

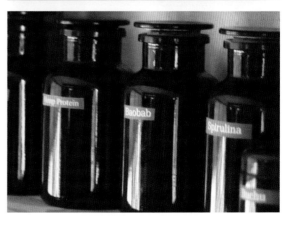

A Superfoodist's Kitchen 17

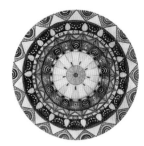

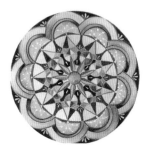

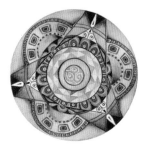

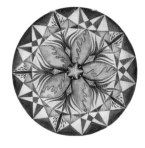

STOCKING THE KITCHEN WITH SUPERFOODS

When you have a good stock of superfoods in your kitchen cupboards, a nutritional meal, snack, or dessert is always close at hand.

Here is a list of superfoods that you will regularly find in our kitchen, along with other ingredients that you will find handy to have when making recipes from this book.

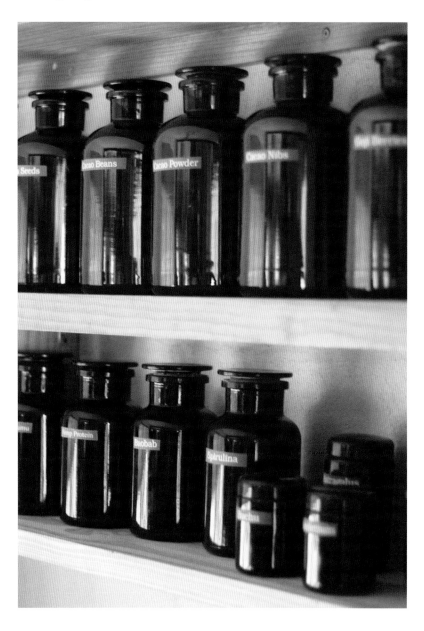

DRIED SUPERFOODS

Baobab powder
Goji berries
Chia seeds
White mulberries
Blue-green algae such as spirulina, chlorella, AFA Klamath crystals
Camu camu powder
Wheatgrass or barleygrass powder
Hemp powder
Shelled hemp seeds
Hemp oil
Coconut oil
Sea vegetables such as nori sheets, kelp powder, kelp noodles, hijiki, kombu, dulse flakes, dulse whole leaf, wakame, arame, sea lettuce
Maca powder
Lucuma powder
Mesquite powder
Yacon root powder
Raw cacao products including raw cacao paste, butter, powder, nibs, and beans
Bee products such as honey, honeycomb, bee pollen, royal jelly, propolis (for the medicine chest)

FRESH SUPERFOODS

Aloe ferox or *Aloe vera* leaves
Berries such as strawberries, blueberries, raspberries, black mulberries, blackberries, gooseberries, and any other wild or exotic berries you can get your hands on
Fresh coconuts or coconut water
Fresh wheatgrass
Fresh sunflower microgreens

MEDICINAL SUPERHERBS

Reishi powder or tincture
Turkey tail mushrooms
Buchu powder or leaf
Sceletium
Ginseng
Foti
Astragalus
Ginkgo biloba
Ashwagandha
Mucuna
Pau d'arco or taheebo

NUTS AND SEEDS

Almonds
Cashews
Macadamia Nuts
Pecans
Brazil Nuts
Hazelnuts
Nut butters
Sunflower seeds
Pumpkin seeds
Flax seeds

SPICES AND SEASONING

Cumin
Cinnamon
Cayenne pepper
Curry powder
Turmeric
Mixed herbs
Kelp powder
Nutmeg
Allspice
Black pepper
Nutritional yeast

SALTS

Himalayan crystal salt
Kalahari Desert salt
Sea salt (non-iodated)
Herbamare vegetable salt

OILS AND VINEGARS

Olive oil
Hemp oil
Apple cider vinegar
Rosendal vinegar
Coconut oil

SWEETENERS AND SWEET DRIED FRUIT

Honey
Maple syrup
Dates
Currants
Raisins
Figs
Vanilla extract
Vanilla powder
Vanilla pods

SAVORY ESSENTIALS

Garlic bulbs
Ginger
Red onions
Chiles
Lemons
Tamari sauce
Tahini
Sundried tomatoes
Black olives
Buckwheat
Oats
Desiccated coconut

FRESH INGREDIENTS FOR JUICING AND SMOOTHIES

Bananas
Apples
Grapefruits
Cucumbers
Celery
Spinach
Parsley
Beetroots
Carrots
Avocados
Mangoes
Passion fruit

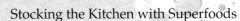

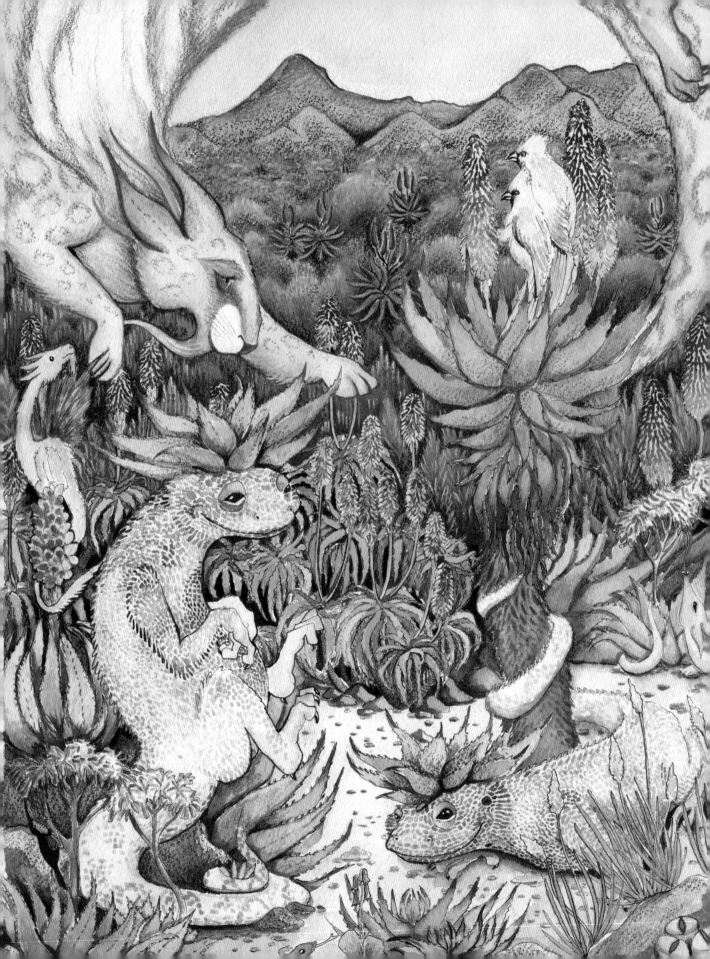

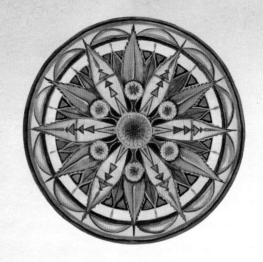

ALOE

GET THE ALOE GLOW

DETOXIFIES * REGENERATES SKIN

ENHANCES IMMUNITY * PROMOTES INTESTINAL HEALTH

REDUCES INFLAMMATION * RESTORES TISSUE ELASTICITY

Where moisture is hidden in a leathery exterior
With energies and remedies, powerful and superior,
A family of Dragons stand guard over the kingdom
Like sentinels on a hill, who will share their wisdom.
Thriving in dry landscapes, as well as green,
The Aloes, in their majesty, stand tall to be seen.
With flowers like fireworks shooting to the sky,
Filled with nectar for creatures that walk and that fly.
A lattice of sugars, minerals, and dew
In their leaves makes a health-giving food just for you:
Healing, hydrating, and smoothing your skin
And your gut—aloe glow, both without and within!

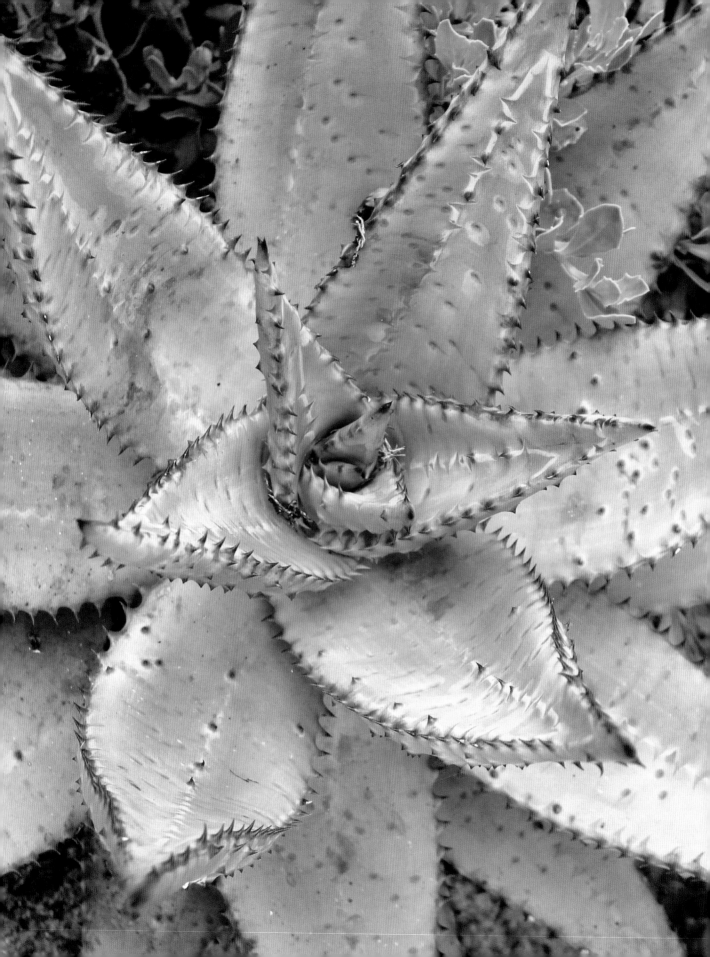

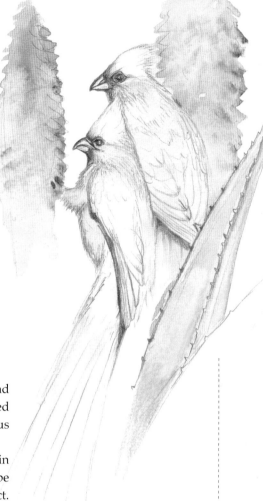

ANCIENT, REVERED SUPERFOOD

The ancient Egyptians revered the healing power of this superfood and bred most of the cultivars we know today. The Essenes also cultivated aloe near the Dead Sea over two thousand years ago. An enormous amount of research has been done on the healing abilities of aloe.

Aloe ferox is our own local superfood! Aloes are experts at living in dry environments, and bring to us the gift of moisture. They can be eaten or applied to the skin, and have a soothing, hydrating effect. Aloe is known to stimulate the production of collagen in the body, which maintains flexibility in the skin, bones, joints, and tissues.

I remember the first time I saw someone put a wedge of aloe into a smoothie. A lightbulb went on in my head! As a child I had always suffered with eczema, and my mom used to have different aloe lotions that she would apply to my skin. While they had some soothing effect, the "Aha!" realization I had when I saw that chunk of aloe go into the blender was this: the key is to moisturize from the inside out, not the other way around!

Aloes are a succulent desert plant that grow in deserts and sub-tropical regions. Their healing power is well known and documented around the globe. *Aloe ferox* is native to southern Africa. We are lucky to have such an abundance of aloes around us. We have wild-harvested aloe leaves from the coasts of Cape Town to the deserts of Botswana, often pulling off on the side of the highway to harvest this plentiful, powerful, and free superfood.

ALOES PROVIDE MEDICINE AND NUTRITION TO HUMANS AND ANIMALS, SUCH AS MOUSEBIRDS, WHO LOVE THEIR SWEET NECTAR, ALIKE.

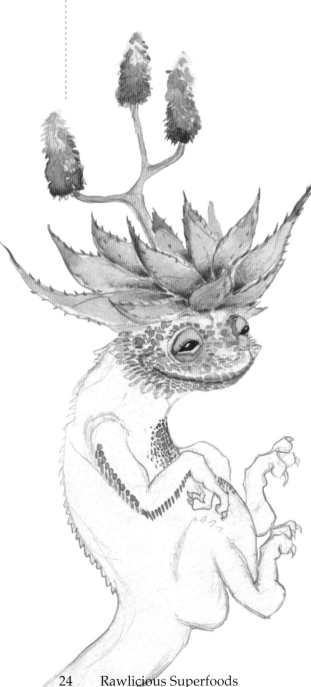

HOW TO IDENTIFY *ALOE VERA* OR *ALOE FEROX*

Aloe ferox

It's easy to spot an *Aloe ferox*. It has a single stem with tough leaves that angle toward the sky and have sharp thorns along the edges. When it flowers, it boasts beautiful red flowering stalks.

Aloe vera

Aloe vera is a stemless or very short-stemmed plant growing 24–40 inches tall. The leaves are thick and fleshy, green to gray-green, with some varieties showing white flecks on their upper and lower stem surfaces. They are softer and less thorny than the *Aloe ferox*.

Aloes are widely available in nurseries, so be sure to plant them in your garden.

HOW WE USE *ALOE FEROX*

The simplest and best way to use aloe is to take a fresh wedge of the inner gel-like substance of *Aloe vera* or *Aloe ferox* and juice or blend it through into your drinks. Fresh aloe leaves are always best, but, if you can't get your hands on fresh leaves, then *Aloe vera* or *Aloe ferox* juices sold in health food stores are also excellent.

We love to wild-harvest aloe. It's easy and fun, but be warned: the leaves have thorns that can bite! Always harvest the bottom leaves, leaving the top ones to grow large. The leaves are ripe when the tips have a slight red blush.

Using a sharp knife, slice through the green skin as close to the base as possible and simply pull the leaf off. The gap left in the plant will seal over and close up very quickly, leaving the plant undamaged. A bright yellow liquid will run out of the cut leaf. These are the aloe bitters, which you simply rinse off before use.

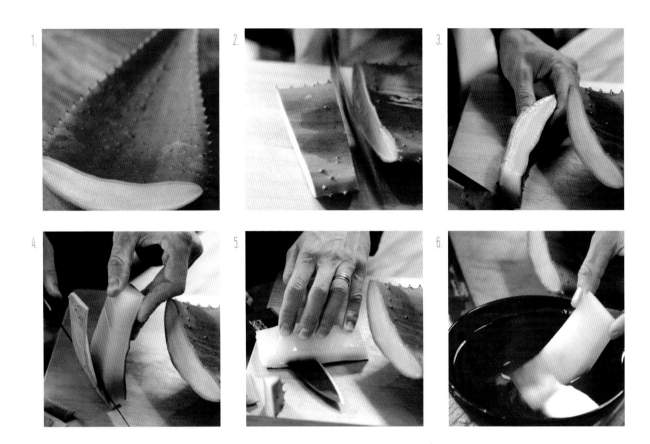

USING *ALOE* DIRECTLY ON YOUR SKIN

Aloe vera is the better type of aloe to use directly on the skin, as it is more liquid. It is great as a simple moisturizer as well as for cuts, grazes, rashes, and burns. Apply the gel from an *Aloe vera* plant directly onto the skin for an instant facelift. (At first it feels all slimy, but within minutes the goodness of the aloe will absorb into your pores!)

WARNINGS

Aloe strongly cleanses the liver, so pregnant women and young children should not use it internally.

THIS IS HOW YOU HARVEST AND PREPARE *ALOE FEROX*. *ALOE VERA* GEL IS ONE OF THE BEST NATURAL TREATMENTS AVAILABLE FOR FIRST-DEGREE AND SECOND-DEGREE SUNBURNS.

THE MAGIC OF ALOE

- DETOXIFIES
- REGENERATES SKIN
- ENHANCES IMMUNITY
- PROMOTES INTESTINAL HEALTH
- REDUCES INFLAMMATION
- RESTORES TISSUE ELASTICITY

The polysaccharides found in aloe have a powerful lubricating effect on the joints, skin, brain, and nervous system. They are immune modulating, strengthening the immune system. They allow the body to overcome viral and fungal infections.

Detoxifies

Aloe is a powerful digestive system cleanser, supporting the colon to release old waste and regain flexibility. It is also a powerful liver cleanser.

Regenerates Skin

Aloe gel can be used topically to treat most skin conditions such as acne, eczema, stings, rashes, sunburns, and wounds. Used regularly, the gel can prevent and even reverse skin damage. Because it stimulates collagen production, it makes your skin look younger, more beautiful, and gives you a natural facelift. Collagen maintains the flexibility in your skin, bones, joints, and tissues.

Enhances immunity

Aloe stimulates the liver into producing glutathione, a key antioxidant in the creation of white blood cells. Glutathione has also been shown to reduce dangerous homocysteine levels when used with vitamins B6, B9, and B12, and folic acid. Acemannan in aloe has also been shown to have powerful anticarcinogenic effects.

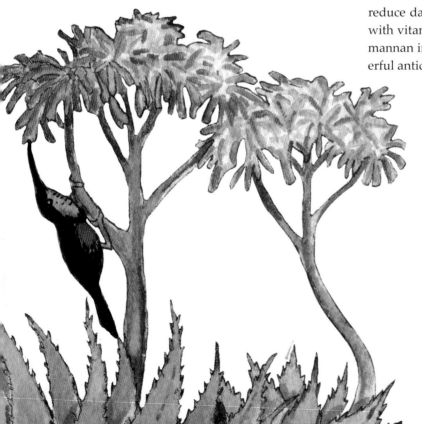

Promotes intestinal health

Aloe is a powerful digestive regenerator and helps with the healing of intestinal disorders such as indigestion, heartburn, hyperacidity, peptic and duodenal ulcers, colitis, and hemorrhoids. Its ability to dissolve mucus helps clear the intestines, allowing better nutrient absorption. It also kills candida and supports healthy friendly bacteria. Aloe polysaccharides are converted in the body to oligosaccharides that attack dangerous organisms such as *E. coli* and *Streptococcus*.

Reduces inflammation

Using aloe topically is widely known to ease inflammation of joints, reducing arthritic pain. But aloe can also be used internally, reducing inflammation throughout the body from the inside out. The mannose polysaccharide in aloe reduces inflammation and is antiviral, antifungal, antiparasitic, and antibacterial. Studies have shown that aloe reduces cholesterol and triglycerides and increases healthy HDL (high-density lipoprotein). The fresh gel has also been shown to normalize blood sugar levels due to its triterpene content.

Restores tissue elasticity—juicy tissues

Aloe contains sulfur similar to MSM (methylsulphonylmethane). It hydrates tissues, reducing collagen damage, hardening of the organs, and wrinkles while restoring elasticity and flexibility.

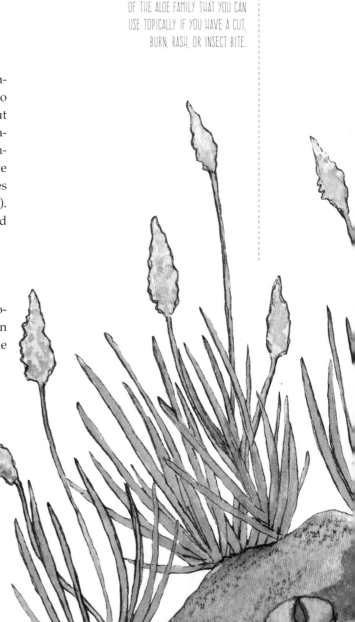

BULBINELLA IS ANOTHER MEMBER OF THE ALOE FAMILY THAT YOU CAN USE TOPICALLY IF YOU HAVE A CUT, BURN, RASH, OR INSECT BITE.

ALOE RECIPES

ALOE CITRUS * ALOE AND GINGER SHOTS

EASY-DRINKING ALOE ALKALIZER * ALOE AND GRAPEFRUIT SKIN CLEANSER

ALOE LEMONADE * ALOE AND MINT DRESSING

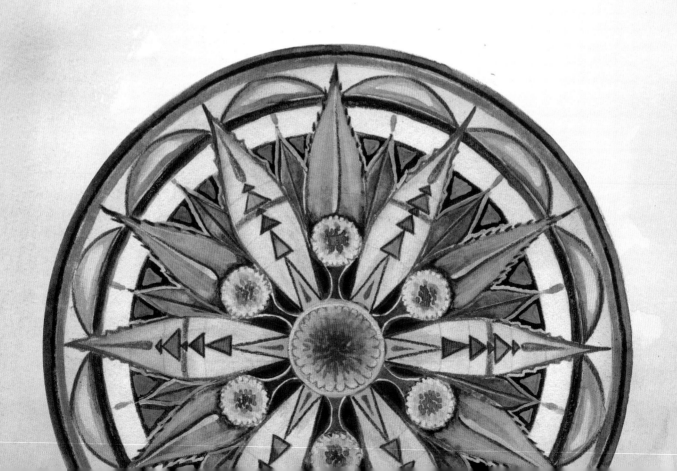

ALOE CITRUS

Vitamin C immune booster

We detoxed by drinking around 25 oz of this drink every day for three days while spending the rest of our time in the hot springs in Kwazulu-Natal.

Makes 2 qt

> 1 qt water
> 2 grapefruits, juiced
> 2 oranges
>
> ½ aloe leaf
> 1 T camu camu powder
> 1 handful goji berries
> 1 handful buchu/mint
> ⅓ inch ginger
> 2 T honey
> 1 passion fruit (optional)

Blend all the ingredients together in a blender.

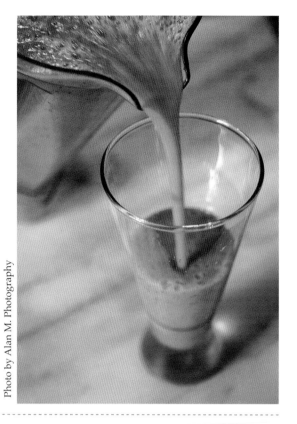

Photo by Alan M. Photography

ALOE AND GINGER SHOTS

Anti-inflammatory

A neat shot of aloe and ginger juice is one of the quickest ways to warm your system on a cold winter's day and to protect yourself from the winter blues and flus.

Makes 2–3 shots

> 1 whole ginger rhizome
> ½ aloe leaf
> 1 lemon

Juice all the ingredients, pour the juice into a shot glass, and knock it back. You can tame the fire of this juice by adding a little apple juice if desired.

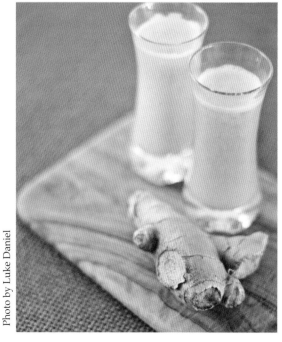

Photo by Luke Daniel

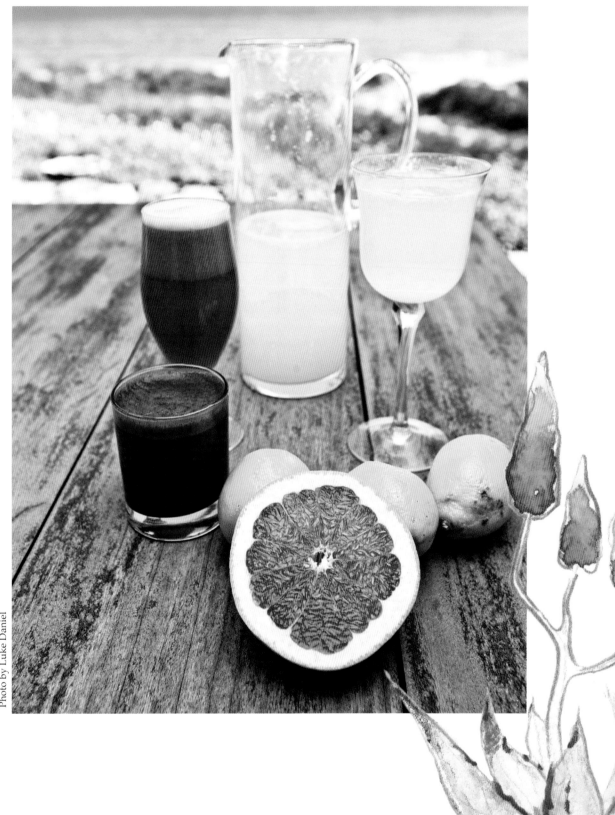

EASY-DRINKING ALOE ALKALIZER

We used to make this juice every morning for about three months when we first transitioned to a high raw diet. The sweet orange juice makes the green powder super palatable and masks any bitterness of the aloe juice.

Juice the oranges and aloe leaf. Stir or blend in the grass powder.

Makes 2 glasses

3 oranges
½ aloe leaf
1 T barleygrass powder,
or wheatgrass powder

ALOE AND GRAPEFRUIT SKIN CLEANSER

Grapefruits are known to help cut cellulite quickly. They contain the enzyme bromelain, which is both anti-inflammatory and skin-cleansing. Combine this with the rejuvenating, collagen-stimulating properties of aloe plus some potent camu camu for extra vitamin C and you've got the best "get-the-aloe-glow" skin tonic!

Juice the grapefruits and the aloe leaf. Stir or blend in the camu camu powder.

Makes 2 glasses

3 grapefruits
½ aloe leaf
1 T camu camu powder

ALOE LEMONADE

Juice the lemon and aloe leaf. Stir in the honey, and slowly pour into the sparkling water.

Makes 1.5 qt

1 lemon
½ aloe leaf
2–3 T honey
1 qt sparkling water

ALOE AND MINT DRESSING

Love your skin inside and out!

This is a delicious salad dressing that will care for your skin from the inside. And it can also be used on the outside.

Blend all the ingredients together. Pour over salads or use on your skin as a face mask, then rinse off.

Makes 2 C

1 avocado
½ C olive oil
1 handful mint
1 wedge aloe, 2 inches
¼ C water
¼ C lemon juice
1 T honey
½ t salt

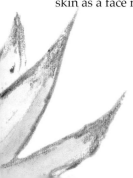

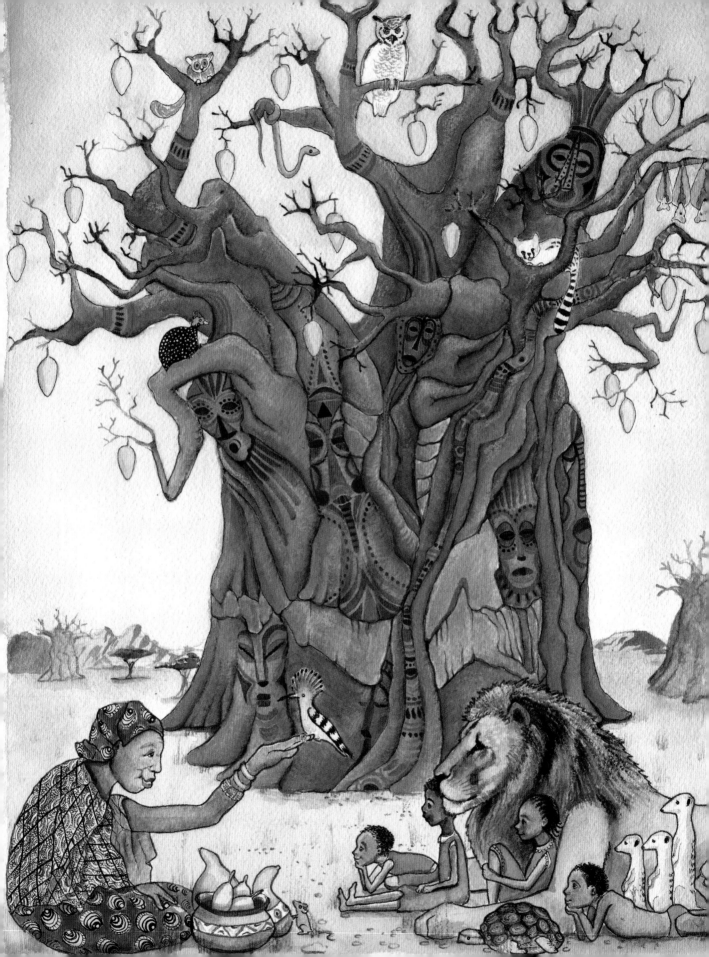

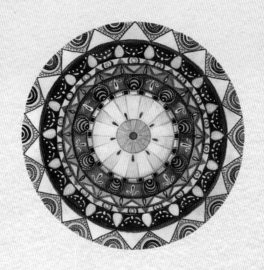

BAOBAB

THE AFRICAN TREE OF LIFE

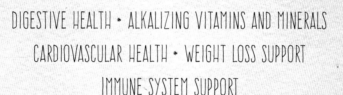

DIGESTIVE HEALTH ✴ ALKALIZING VITAMINS AND MINERALS
CARDIOVASCULAR HEALTH ✴ WEIGHT LOSS SUPPORT
IMMUNE SYSTEM SUPPORT

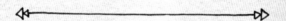

Grandmother Africa, all wrapped in story,
A crown of fruit-laden branches her glory,
The voices of ancestors guide her in whispers,
To care for the generations, our brothers and sisters,
To remind us that we are all part of the earth,
In a community, a cycle of life, death and birth.
This continuum of growth, which we all travel through
Includes all creation, and all points of view.
The baobab is also a community tree,
Providing food, shade, and shelter for many, you see.
So listen to Grandmother, she's listening too,
To the voice of the earth, and the old and the new.
Our lives are like melodies, part of a great song,
Which reminds us of creation, and where we belong.

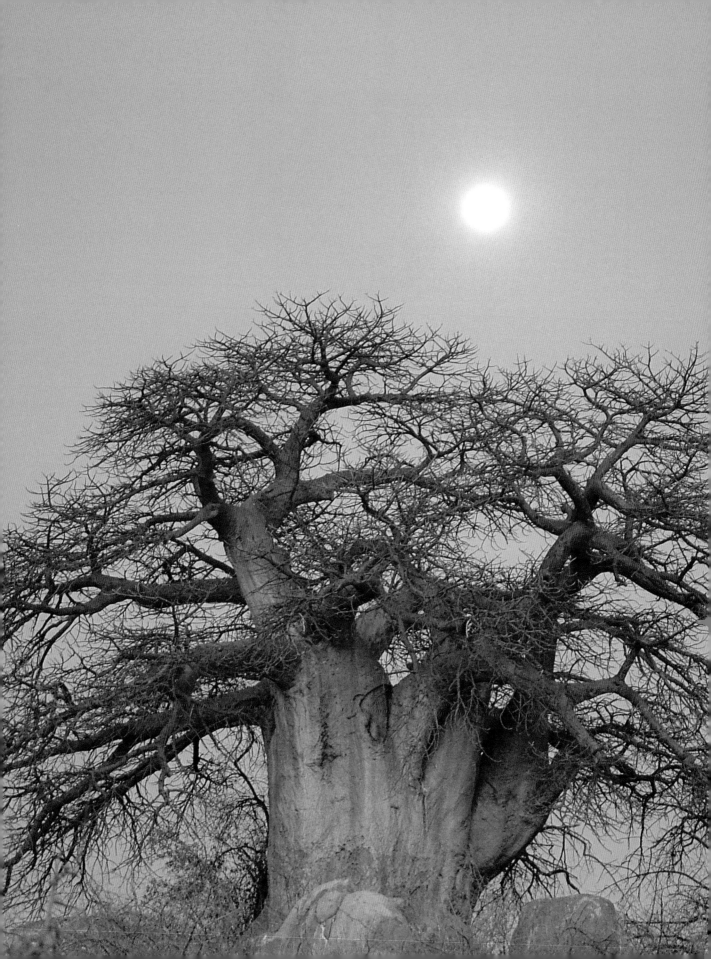

ANCIENT, REVERED SUPERFOOD

In our search for African superfoods, it didn't take long before we stumbled across the baobab. The baobab has been used medicinally by traditional cultures for centuries and is steeped in traditional folklore.

Known as the upside-down tree, the cream-of-tartar tree, or the African tree of life, the ancient baobab gifts us with its exceptional fruit. The beautiful, heavy, white flowers of the baobab tree are pollinated by nocturnal fruit bats. The large green or brownish fruits resemble gourd-like capsules of around 5–6 inches in length. These capsules contain a soft, whitish fruit pulp that has the appearance of powdery bread and kidney-shaped seeds. Unlike other fruit, baobab dries naturally on the branches of the tree. The fruit is wild-harvested by collecting the pods from the trees. The powder has a unique tangy taste described as caramel pear with subtle tones of grapefruit.

The baobab must be one of Africa's most magical trees. We have climbed a tree that is estimated to be two thousand years old, and that still produces fruit.

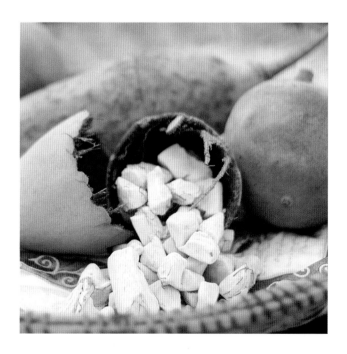

ALL PARTS OF THE BAOBAB TREE HAVE MEDICINAL PROPERTIES ACCORDING TO TRADITIONAL FOLKLORE.

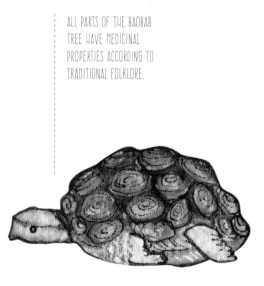

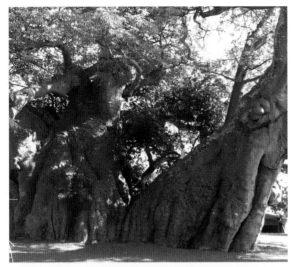

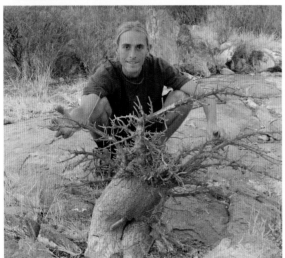

The Sunland Big Baobab in the Limpopo province in South Africa is famous for being the widest of its species in the world. When baobabs become a thousand years old, they begin to hollow out inside. This one even has a bar inside where we blended up a decadent baobab and cacao smoothie.

Baobab fruit is exceptionally rich in antioxidants and essential minerals and has been used medicinally by traditional cultures for centuries. Of particular interest is the use of the baobab fruit and seeds to treat dysentery. It is also used to make a solution for the treatment of dehydration. For centuries, the women of Africa have turned to the baobab tree as a source of natural well-being, to benefit their skin, hair, and general health. In Sudan, a refreshing drink called gubdi is made with the fruit pulp and cold water.

HOW WE USE BAOBAB

The creamy baobab powder melts in the mouth when eaten and has a unique, pleasant flavor with a mild, tangy taste. It is the original sherbet. We use it in juices, smoothies, and other drinks or as a thickener in desserts or sauces.

THE SUNLAND BAOBAB MAY BE BIG, BUT THIS BABY BAOBAB WE FOUND ON KHUBU ISLAND IN BOTSWANA IS *SO CUTE!*

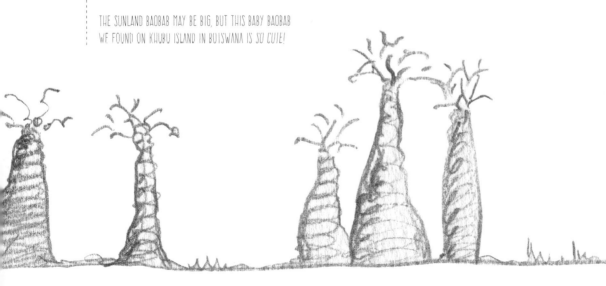

THE MAGIC OF BAOBAB

- DIGESTIVE HEALTH
- ALKALIZING VITAMINS AND MINERALS
- CARDIOVASCULAR HEALTH
- WEIGHT LOSS SUPPORT
- IMMUNE SYSTEM SUPPORT

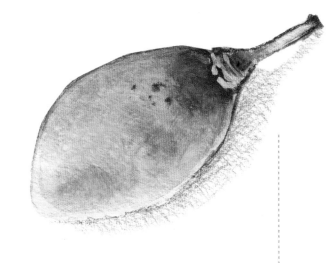

BAOBAB FRUIT IS AN EXCELLENT SOURCE OF PECTINS, CALCIUM, VITAMIN C, AND IRON.

Digestive health

Baobab contains higher levels of pectin dietary fiber than many other fruits, including apples, peaches, apricots, and bananas. It is also a prebiotic and helps to feed the good bacteria in the gut, supporting overall digestive health.

Alkalizing vitamins and minerals

Baobab contains higher levels of calcium than milk, and is far easier to absorb and digest, allowing the body to maintain strong bones and teeth. Baobab is an excellent source of thiamin (vitamin B1), vitamin C, and vitamin B6, which contribute to the processes that yield energy in the body and reduce tiredness and fatigue. Baobab is also a significant source of iron, potassium, and magnesium, all of which are important alkalizing minerals to promote correct body pH.

Cardiovascular health

Pectin is the main source of fiber in baobab, and has been reported to play a role in reducing LDL (low-density lipoprotein) cholesterol.

Weight loss support

The high levels of fiber in baobab means it is naturally low in calories, assisting in weight loss.

Immune system support

Baobab fruit powder has more than double the antioxidants of pomegranates and cranberries, and more than three times that of blueberries. Baobab contains up to ten times more vitamin C than oranges. Coupled with its high essential mineral profile, this makes baobab a great immune system support food.

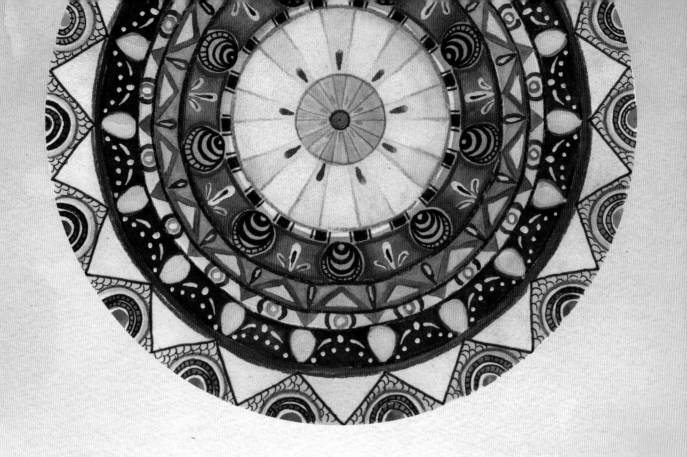

BAOBAB RECIPES

BAO JUICE ∗ IN-THE-BAOBAB CACAO SMOOTHIE

BAO BEER ∗ BAO-MAYO ∗ BAO SORBET ∗ THE ORIGINAL SHERBET

BAO JUICE

Calcium-rich alkalizer

Makes 8 ounces, dilute with the same quantity of water to make 16 ounces

> 2 apples
> ½ cucumber
> 2–4 spinach leaves
> ½ lemon
> 1 T baobab powder
> 1 t wheatgrass or barleygrass powder (optional)

Juice the apples, cucumber, spinach, and lemon. Add the baobab powder and grass powder, and stir or blend together.

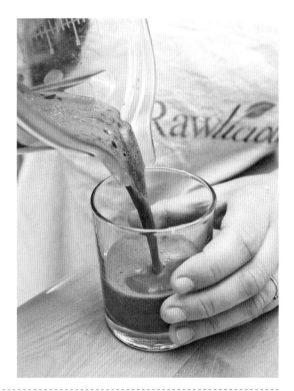

IN-THE-BAOBAB CACAO SMOOTHIE

Energizing bao-cacao combo

Makes 1 qt

> 3 C water
> ¼ C cashews
> 1 banana
> ¼ C baobab powder
> ¼ C cacao powder
> ¼ C dates
> ⅛ C yacon powder
> ⅛ C coconut oil
> ¼ t vanilla extract or seeds from 1 vanilla pod
> ¼ C cacao nibs (optional)

Blend all the ingredients together and enjoy.

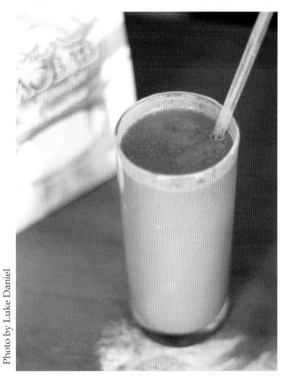

Photo by Luke Daniel

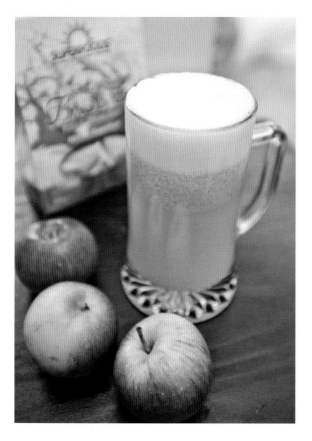

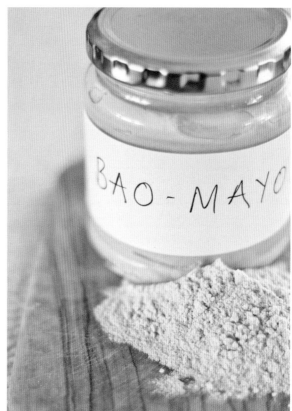

Photos by Luke Daniel

BAO BEER

Baobab-ginger digestive

Makes 1 qt

  2 lemons
  2 apples
  2-inch piece of ginger
  3 C sparkling water
  2 t baobab powder, heaping
  2 T honey

Juice the lemons, apples, and ginger. Add remaining ingredients and blend.

BAO-MAYO

Prebiotic bao-naise

When we discovered this "mayonnaise" recipe, it was a revelation. We quickly dubbed it bao-mayo or bao-naise.

Makes ½ qt

  ¾ C olive oil
  2 T apple cider vinegar
  2 T baobab powder, heaping
  1 garlic clove
  1 t honey
  ½ t salt
  ¾ C water

Blend all the ingredients together except the water. Add the water last and blend on high until the mixture thickens.

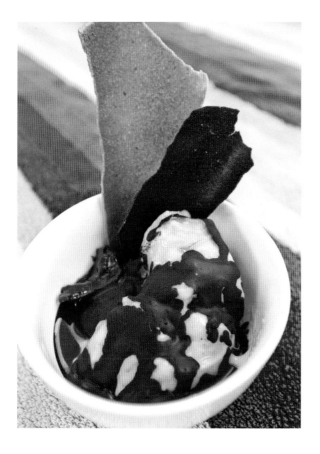

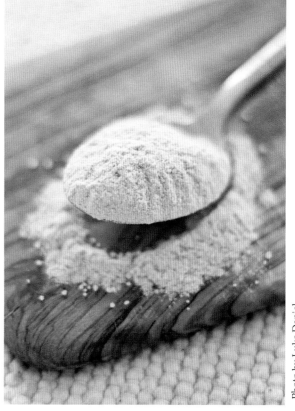

BAO SORBET

Immune-boosting bao-camu sorbet or popsicles

Serves 2–3

> 1 pineapple, peeled
> 1 apple, peeled
> 1 lemon, peeled
> 1 T baobab powder
> 1 t camu camu powder
> 1 T honey

Freeze the fruit. Blend all the ingredients together in a power blender and refreeze. Alternatively, you can juice the fruit, blend in the baobab, camu camu powder, and honey, and freeze in popsicle molds.

THE ORIGINAL SHERBET

Sugar-free healthy sherbet

Makes 2 oz

> 2 T baobab powder
> 1 T camu camu powder
> 1 T xylitol

Mix all ingredients together and enjoy.

You can make as much of this sherbet as you please by increasing the ingredients according to the ratio above.

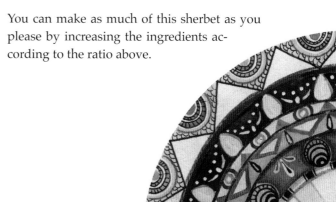

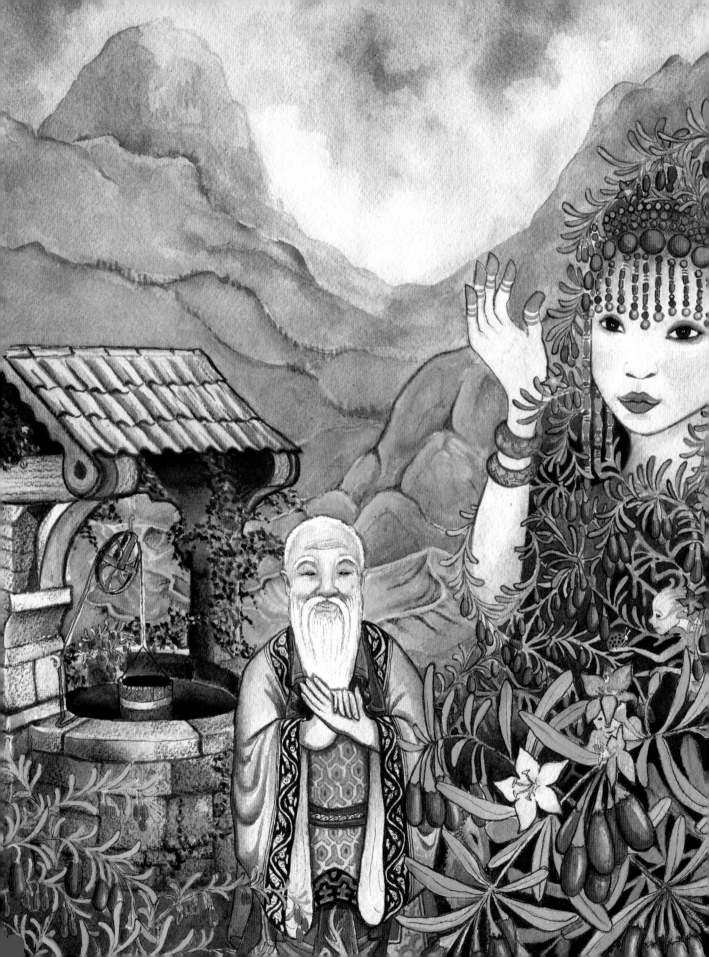

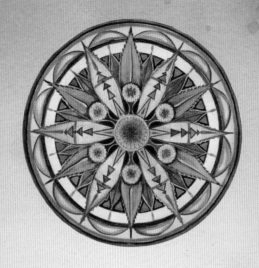

GOJI BERRIES

LONGEVITY SUPERFOOD

ADAPTOGEN JING BUILDER • COMPLETE PROTEIN SOURCE

VITAMIN AND MINERAL RICH • IMPROVES EYESIGHT • YOUTHENING

IMMUNE BOOSTING • DIGESTIVE SUPPORT • CARDIOVASCULAR HEALTH

Once upon a time amongst ancient hills
There was a temple where monks used to pray
Some people who observed the monks over many years,
Noticed that they had hardly aged a day.
"What are they doing? To whom do they pray?
Is it some deity that halts their decay?"
'Til they realized that the monks drank from a well
That was built near the temple, all covered in vines:
Goji vines, off of which goji berries fell
Infusing the water down deep in the well.
A living vibration that speaks to our cells
We realize the source from which our life force wells
A question of Time as illusion or truth
Ancient wisdom, fountain of youth.

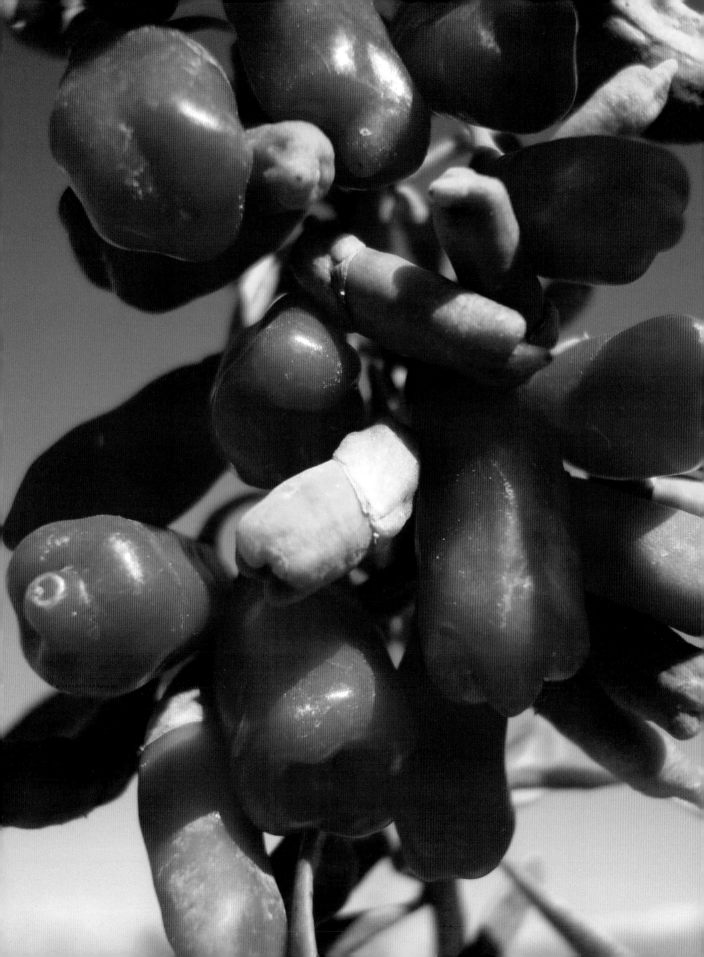

ANCIENT, REVERED SUPERFOOD

The goji berry has been highly regarded for centuries as a foremost nutritional and botanical medicine in China. Gojis have been grown in Tibet, China, and Mongolia for an estimated five thousand years, and have been recognized as a superfood by the Tibetan School of medicine for 2,500 years.

In China, the spirit of the goji is often represented as a young, strong woman, as the Chinese strongly believe that gojis extend life. Just take the example of Li Qing Yuen, one of the best documented cases of extreme longevity. He lived to the age of 252 years (1678–1930) and is said to have consumed goji berries daily. In Chinese medicine they are considered a "tonic" herb, meaning that daily use has a cumulative effect over time.

We were first introduced to goji berries at a holistic trade fair. The salesman raved about them and encouraged us to taste them. We were surprised that something so healthy was so delicious. The goji berry's Latin name, *Lycium*, comes from the root meaning "school of learning." Chinese herbalists believe that the berry can link one into the teachings of Chinese medicine, generally making one more aware of health. Gojis were the first superfood we were introduced to, and I believe they had a subtle yet powerful guiding effect on us, helping us to embark on our journey into health education.

Since then, we've been eating gojis almost daily for over a decade. We probably eat gojis more regularly than any other superfood.

Having been to the Tibetan plateau and seen the harsh, dry environment where gojis grow, it is no wonder that they are also known as an adaptogenic superfood, assisting us to adapt to stressors. We've even seen goji berries growing off the edge of an ocean cliff in the Western Cape in South Africa.

IT IS SAID IN CHINA THAT EATING A HANDFUL OF GOJI BERRIES EACH DAY WILL MAKE ONE HAPPY FOR THE ENTIRE DAY. SUCH A PRACTICE HAS A CUMULATIVE EFFECT. EVENTUALLY, YOU CAN'T STOP SMILING!

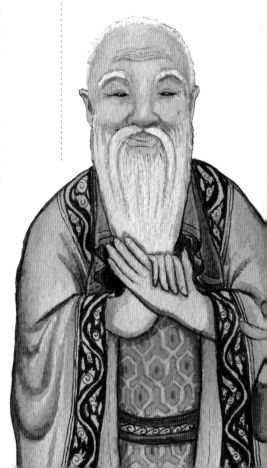

THE MAGIC OF GOJI BERRIES

- ADAPTOGEN JING BUILDER
- COMPLETE PROTEIN SOURCE
- VITAMIN AND MINERAL RICH
- IMPROVES EYESIGHT
- YOUTHENING
- IMMUNE BOOSTING
- DIGESTIVE SUPPORT
- CARDIOVASCULAR HEALTH

GOJI'S BOTANICAL NAME IS *LYCIUM,*
WHICH MEANS "SCHOOL OF LEARNING."

Adaptogen jing builder

Gojis are an adaptogen, meaning they invigorate and strengthen the body and help it deal with stress by supporting the adrenal glands. According to Chinese medicine, they boost kidney and adrenal jing energy, enhancing stamina, longevity, and sexual energy.

Complete protein source

Goji berries contain eighteen kinds of amino acids, the building blocks of protein, including all eight essential amino acids. These body-building proteins are also brain supportive, including the serotonin-producing tryptophan.

Vitamin and mineral rich

Gojis are rich in twenty-one trace minerals, of which the main ones are zinc, iron, copper, calcium, germanium, selenium, and phosphorus. They are also packed with vitamins B1, B2, and B6, which boost energy.

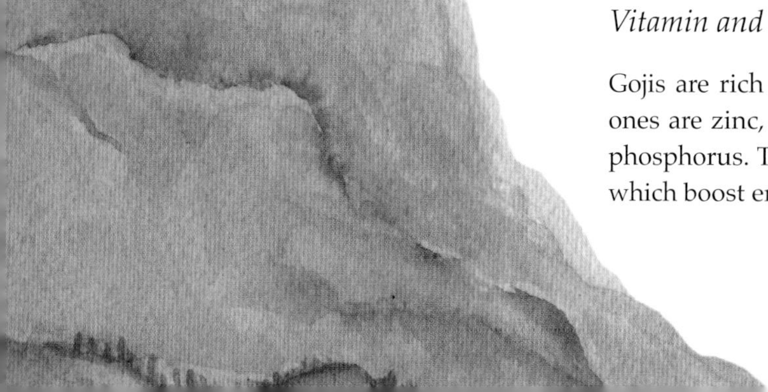

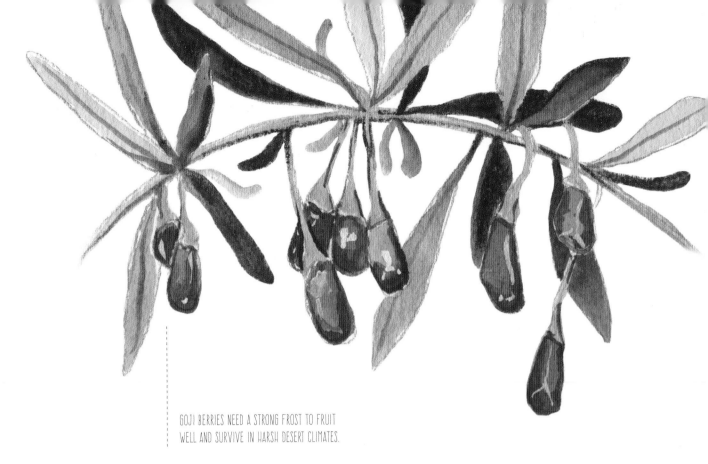

GOJI BERRIES NEED A STRONG FROST TO FRUIT WELL AND SURVIVE IN HARSH DESERT CLIMATES.

Improves eyesight

Goji berries are very high in antioxidants. They are one of the best sources of carotenoids of all known common foods and plants on earth, and contain betacarotene and zeaxanthin. This high antioxidant value protects your DNA from free radical damage. Gojis' incredibly high zeaxanthin and lutein content protects and improves eyesight.

Youthening

The sesquiterpenoids in gojis have powerful anti-inflammatory properties and increase the glandular production of HGH (human growth hormone), our master youthening hormone. They are the only known food that is a confirmed secretagogue, boosting HGH. Increasing your body's carotenoid content has also been shown to increase your maximal lifespan potential (MLSP).

Immune boosting

Goji berries contain polysaccharides (LBPs, or *Lycium barbarum* polysaccharides), which have been demonstrated to strongly fortify the immune system.

Digestive support

In China, gojis are added to almost everything eaten—soups, stews, salads, and teas. They do this because gojis stimulate the release of digestive juices, which helps you digest food better. The betaine in gojis also enhance digestion.

Cardiovascular health

Gojis increase our production of superoxide dismutase (SOD), which prevents cholesterol from oxidizing and attaching to arterial walls.

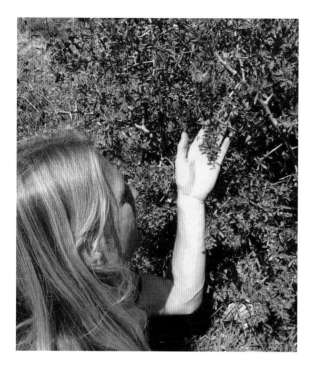

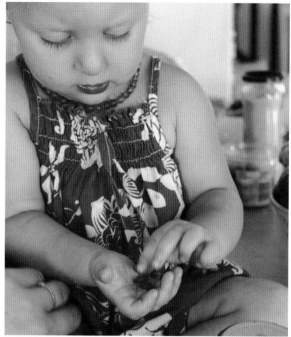

Photo by Luke Daniel

QUALITY IS KEY!

Most gojis are grown in China and may contain high levels of pesticides, be sprayed with the toxic preservative sulfur dioxide, and even be dyed redder with chemicals. Any potential benefits are likely to be entirely neutralized or negated by such dangerous chemical additives.

Make sure you buy only certified organic gojis, certified by a reputable organization in the United States or Europe. Fake Chinese organic certificates are all too common!

HOW WE USE GOJI BERRIES

Goji berries have a unique, slightly sweet taste reminiscent of cranberries and raisins.

We start our day off with a glass of goji water. We often add gojis to our smoothies or sprinkle them over our breakfast. They are delicious added into soups and salads. They also mix well with other dried fruits, seeds, and nuts for your own blood-sugar stabilizing trail mix. They are the perfect sweet treat. Take the time to try out our Hearty Goji Balls recipe—they are unbelievably addictive.

The typical daily intake range suggested by Chinese herbalists is between 0.25 and 1 oz (8 and 30 g) per day. A minimum of 0.35–0.5 oz (10–15 g, a small handful) of the fruit should be eaten daily for maintenance, and dosages as high as 1.5 oz (45 g) per day are suggested for tonic adaptogenic effect.

Children love to snack on gojis! Our young daughter, Katara, picks the soft gojis out of our goji water in the morning.

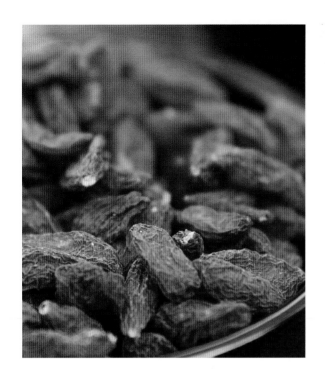

THERE ARE OVER 100 DIFFERENT SPECIES OF GOJIS ALL OVER THE WORLD. ONE EVEN GROWS NATURALLY IN SOUTH AFRICA!

GROW YOUR OWN! HIGH-QUALITY GOJI BERRIES ARE FULL OF VIABLE SEEDS. PLANT THEM IN YOUR GARDEN AND GROW YOUR OWN FRUIT.

THE ORAC SCALE (OXYGEN RADICAL ABSORBANCE CAPACITY) WAS DEVELOPED AT TUFTS UNIVERSITY AND MEASURES THE ANTIOXIDANT VALUES IN FOOD.

COMPARE THE ANTIOXIDANTS!

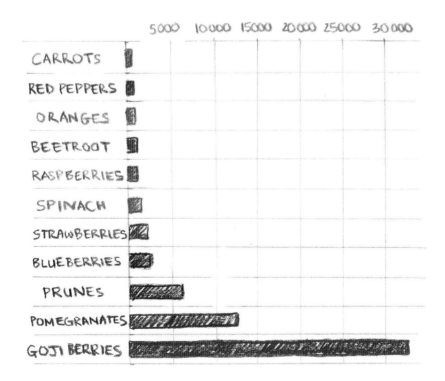

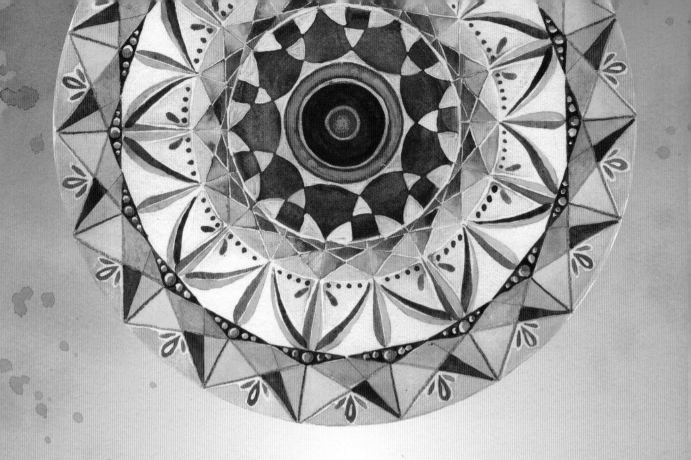

GOJI BERRY RECIPES

GOJI INFUSIONS * GOJI WINTER CITRUS * YUMMY GUMMYBERRY GOJI JUICE
GOJI ICE/POPSICLES * GET-UP-AND-GO GOJI GRANOLA * GOJI TOMATO SOUP
HEARTY GOJI BALLS * GOJI AND ORANGE CARROT CAKE

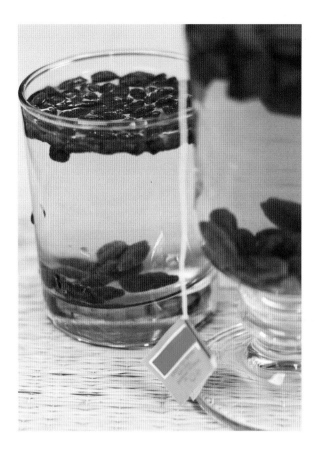

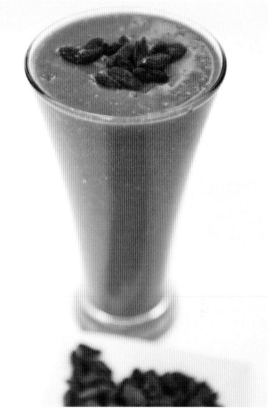

Photos by Luke Daniel

GOJI INFUSIONS

Live-long goji water

We start most mornings with this drink.

> *1 handful goji berries in 1–2 C warm or cold water*

Infuse the gojis in the water for five minutes. Remember to eat the softened gojis left at the bottom of the glass or use them in a smoothie.

Goji digestive tea

Add a handful of goji berries to your cup or pot of green tea (or your favorite tea—buchu or rooibos also work well). Add honey to taste.

Tip: Green tea dilates your cells. Adding gojis to your tea helps drive their goodness into your cells.

GOJI WINTER CITRUS

Season-change immune booster

This drink is loaded with fruits high in vitamin C, such as oranges, guavas, camu camu powder, and of course gojis, and is great for boosting the immune system as the seasons change.

Makes 1.25 qt

> 2 C water
> 3 guavas
> 1 orange
> ½ lemon
> ¼ C goji berries
> 1 T camu camu powder
> 2 T honey

Blend all the ingredients together.

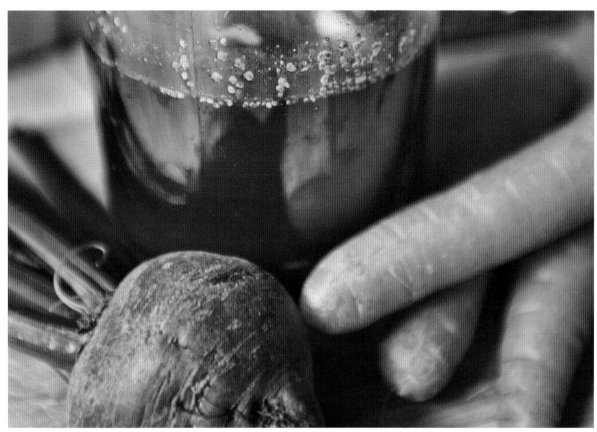

Photo by Luke Daniel

YUMMY GUMMYBERRY GOJI JUICE
Super-sight power juice

Makes 2 C

> ½ *pineapple or 2 apples*
> 2 *carrots*
> 1 *beetroot*
> ½ *lemon*
> ¼ *C gojis soaked in 1 C water*

Goji berries are among the highest sources of carotenoids of all known foods. They contain betacarotene and zeaxanthin, which help improve eyesight. Combine them with other betacarotene-rich vegetables, such as carrots and beetroots, and enjoy this bright, rejuvenating elixir.

Juice the pineapple or apples, carrots, beetroot, and lemon. Put the soaked goji berries through the juicer. Keep the goji soak water and add it to the juice.

GOJI ICE / POPSICLES
Take the yummy gummyberry goji juice recipe and set into ice cubes or popsicles. To be enjoyed by children and adults alike!

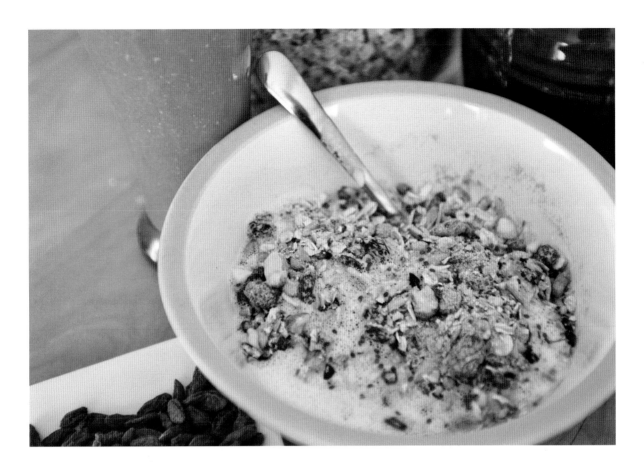

GET-UP-AND-GO GOJI GRANOLA

Make a big jar of this ahead of time so it's quick to get up and get going with this delicious, healthy breakfast cereal.

Pulse the oats, almonds, and sunflower seeds in a food processor until the ingredients are roughly chopped. Put the chopped nuts and seeds into a mixing bowl and add the goji berries, chia seeds, currants or raisins, white mulberries, cacao nibs, lucuma powder, and hemp seeds. Mix together and store in a glass jar.

Spoon into individual breakfast bowls and add a nut or seed milk of your choice. Add a generous dollop of honey to sweeten, and enjoy. This is a very filling breakfast.

2 C raw oats
1 C almonds
1 C sunflower seeds
½ C goji berries
½ C chia seeds
½ C currants or raisins
½ C white mulberries
½ C cacao nibs
¼ C lucuma powder
¼ C hemp seeds

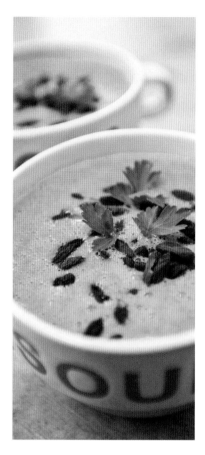

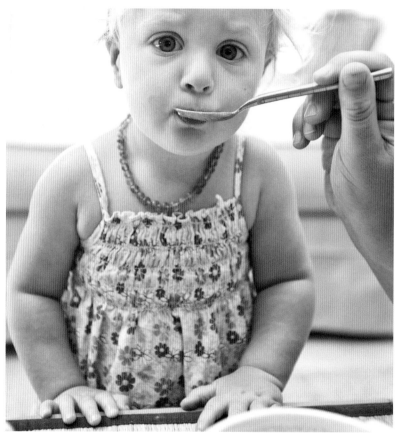

Photos by Luke Daniel

GOJI TOMATO SOUP

Makes 1.5 qt

    3 C hot water
    6 tomatoes
    ½ avocado
    ⅓ C gojis, soaked
    ¼ red onion
    1½ T miso
    2 cloves garlic
    ½ t salt
    ¼ t black pepper

This has been one of Katara's favorite first foods. A simple tomato soup zooped up with goji berries—she loves it.

Blend all ingredients until smooth and creamy.

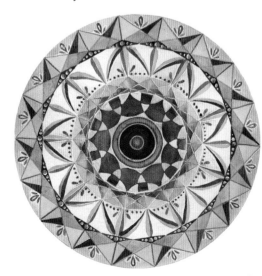

54   **Rawlicious Superfoods**

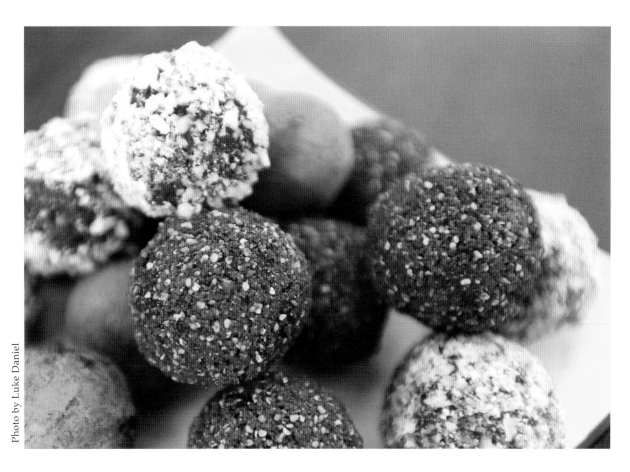

Photo by Luke Daniel

HEARTY GOJI BALLS

Grind goji berries up into a powder in a power blender. They will get sticky, but this is what gives the balls their chewy taste, so go with it!

Blend the dates with half a cup of the soak water into a date jam.

In a food processor, grind your almonds until they reach a crumbly consistency. Set two tablespoons ground almonds aside for rolling the balls in later. Add all the ingredients together, including the date jam, and pulse in the food processor until well combined into a doughy consistency. Roll into balls and coat in ground almonds. For the chocolate version, add the cacao powder to the mixture in the food processor, and decorate with ground gojis or cacao powder.

Tip: When rolling the mixture into balls, dip your fingers in water—the mixture won't stick to your fingers as much.

Makes 15–18 balls

Version 1: without chocolate

> *1 C goji berries*
> *1 C pitted dates, soaked*
> *¾ C almonds, ground fine*
> *½ C lucuma powder*
> *1 t vanilla powder*
> *½ t salt*
> *½ C water*

Version 2: with chocolate

> *Add ½ C cacao powder*

Decorating variations:

> *2 T almonds, ground*
> *2 T cacao powder*
> *a handful of gojis, ground*

Goji Berry Recipes   55

Serves 10–12

For the cake mixture:

> 1 C pitted dates, soaked
> ¼ C water
> 3 C carrots, grated
> 1 C desiccated coconut
> 1 C pecans, chopped
> ½ C raisins
> ¼ C goji berries
> ¼ C chia seeds
> ⅛ C cacao butter, melted
> juice of 1 orange
> 1 t nutmeg
> 1 t allspice
> 1 t cinnamon
> zest of 1 lemon
> pinch salt

For the icing:

> 2 C cashews
> ½ C water
> ¼ C honey
> ⅛ C lucuma powder
> ⅛ C cacao butter
> 1 T lemon juice
> 1 T vanilla extract
> ¼ t salt

GOJI AND ORANGE CARROT CAKE

I love this cake recipe. It has a delicious, different flavor. But the best of all is that you can shape and mold the cake mixture by hand into almost any shape, without the use of a cake tin, and then ice it. I used this mixture to make Katara's first birthday cake—a cake in the shape of a wishing well with a cupcake with a birthday candle. I've used this mixture to make a doll cake for a friend's daughter and to shape a "5" and a "0" for another friend's 50th. It's so versatile and so fun once you get started. Depending on the size of the cake you want to make, you may have to double or even quadruple the recipe. The plain white icing recipe below can be dyed using beetroot juice to make pink icing, spirulina to make green icing, a touch of turmeric to make yellow icing, and so on. Get creative and have fun decorating your cake.

For the cake mixture:

Blend the dates with the soak water. Place all the ingredients together in a bowl and mix well by hand. Place on a cake plate and mold into the desired shape.

For the icing:

Blend all the icing ingredients in a power blender until smooth. Ice your cake and decorate with more goji berries and pecans. Or have fun creating different colored icings and decorating with a piping bag using virtually any design!

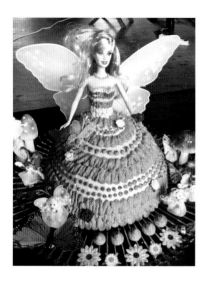

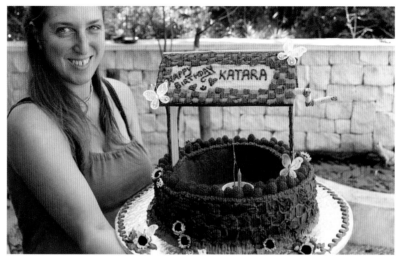

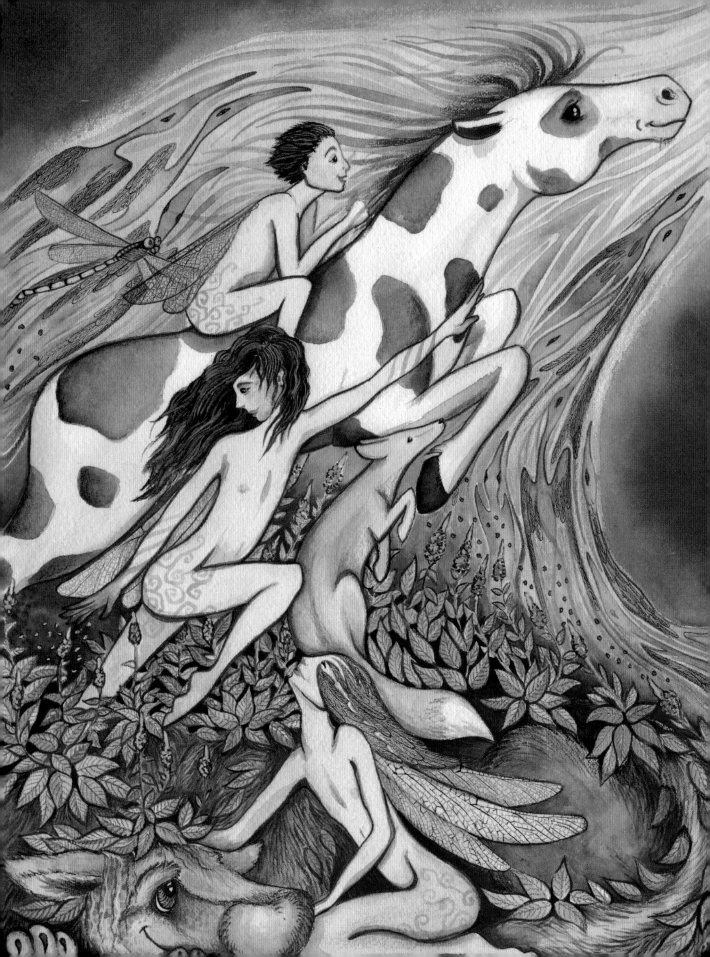

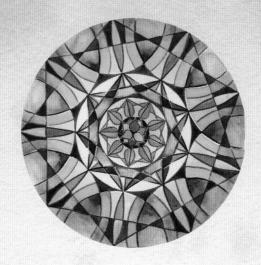

CHIA

OMEGA-3 POWER

———— ✑ ————

BRAIN HEALTH ✲ DIGESTIVE HEALTH ✲ ANTI-INFLAMMATORY
ATHLETIC ENDURANCE, FLEXIBILITY, AND FITNESS ✲ BODY-BUILDING PROTEIN
WEIGHT LOSS ✲ BLOOD SUGAR STABILIZER ✲ CARDIOVASCULAR HEALTH ✲ LONGEVITY

———— ✑ ————

Shooting up skyward on swift wings and feet
The creatures of chia are light, fast, and fleet.
Chia's full of energy that can make your feet fly,
You're the fastest of runners, you're nimble and spry.
First a pretty purple flower, and then small speckled seeds
Which are filled with good oils that will give us that speed.
The chia plant, remember, grows from the ground,
And that is where the Chia Monster can be found—
A big earthy fellow who makes green things sprout.
You'll definitely know when he has been about,
As you'll see little buds peeking out from the rim
Of big furry pawprints that were left there by him!
So it's taught, to grow upward like springtime green shoots,
And levitate high, it must come from your roots!

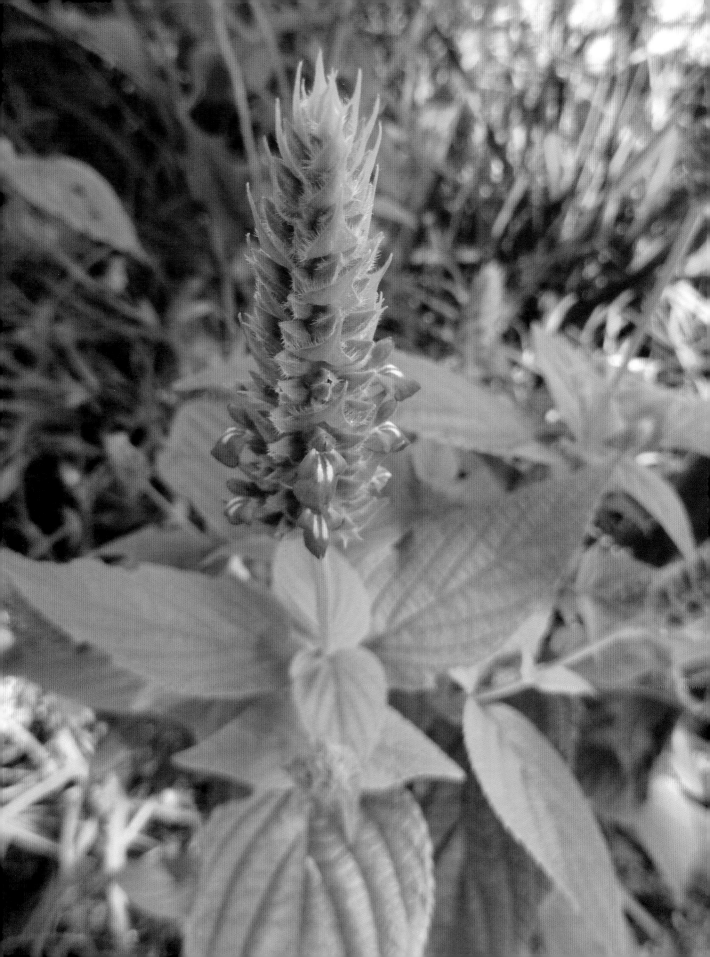

ANCIENT, REVERED SUPERFOOD

Chia literally means "strength" in Mayan, and has over three thousand years of history as an ancient, revered crop. As with many other superfoods, chia was considered more valuable than gold by the Aztecs. The seeds were used as a mega-energy food, especially by the running messengers, who would carry a small pouch of it with them.

Chia is a plant of the sage family. It sends forth purple flowers. The flowers develop into seeds, and it is the seeds of the chia plant that we eat. They are a fantastic source of energy and are known as "the runner's food."

Chia's spectacular nutritional profile makes it a near complete food. It provides essential proteins, fats, and carbohydrates as well as a wide array of vitamins, minerals, and antioxidants. It brings a levitation-like lightness to your step. Its high omega-3 content brings focus and clarity. Perhaps it's because it helps to clear the colon of old waste and unwanted habits that it is so good at making us feel *light*!

Once you start to use chia, its applications unfurl and sprout just as the seed does, revealing itself as a treasure in the budding superfoodist's kitchen.

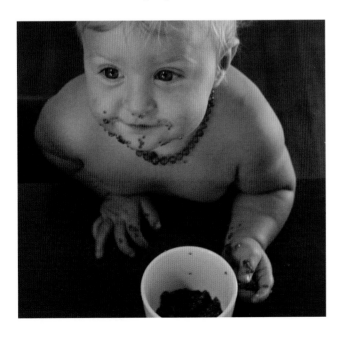

I CAN SCARCELY REMEMBER WHAT WE USED TO EAT FOR BREAKFAST BEFORE WE DISCOVERED CHIA, IT HAS BECOME SUCH A STAPLE IN OUR LIVES.

THE MAGIC OF CHIA

- BRAIN HEALTH
- DIGESTIVE HEALTH
- ANTI-INFLAMMATORY
- ATHLETIC ENDURANCE, FLEXIBILITY, AND FITNESS
- BODY-BUILDING PROTEIN
- WEIGHT LOSS
- BLOOD SUGAR STABILIZER
- CARDIOVASCULAR HEALTH
- LONGEVITY

Brain health—brain food

Chia contains high levels of omega-3 oils. Omega-3s are already well known to support brain development. A number of studies show that reduced intake of omega-3 fatty acids is associated with increased risk of age-related cognitive decline, including Alzheimer's disease. Scientists believe the omega-3 fatty acid DHA protects against Alzheimer's disease and dementia.

Digestive health

The soluble, fiber-rich gel in chia soothes the digestive system and slows the release of sugars into the bloodstream, stabilizing blood sugar levels. Chia is also an excellent colon cleanser and clears out the digestive tract so that you absorb more nutrients and eliminate waste more efficiently.

Anti-inflammatory

Chia is one of the highest plant-based sources of omega-3 EFA (essential fatty acids), outperforming even flaxseed. The excellent ratio of omega-3 to omega-6 of 3:2 makes it a great anti-inflammatory food. EFAs are important for the respiration of vital organs, yet the human body is unable to manufacture them; they must be obtained through diet.

Athletic endurance, flexibility, and fitness

The combination of essential fats, fiber, and protein make chia an excellent food for improving endurance and fitness. It also has the ability to help keep the body hydrated and electrolytes balanced. Its high antioxidants and EFAs help to maintain flexibility in the joints.

Body-building protein

Chia seeds are a near-complete source of protein, containing nineteen amino acids. They contain twice the amount of protein found in almost all other seeds or grains. All essential amino acids except taurine are present and appropriately balanced, making chia seeds an excellent protein source for athletes and vegetarians alike.

Weight loss and blood sugar stabilizer

Chia is known as a dieter's dream food, as it bulks up meals with its low-calorie nutrient density without altering flavor. It makes you feel fuller for longer, reducing food cravings and keeping blood sugar stable.

Cardiovascular health

Clinical evidence of the benefits of omega-3 is strongest for heart disease and problems that contribute to heart disease. Several clinical studies suggest that diets rich in omega-3 fatty acids lower blood pressure in people with hypertension.

Longevity

The potent antioxidants in chia naturally preserve the sensitive omega-3 oils and provide anti-aging benefits. With five times the calcium of milk, plus boron, a trace mineral that helps transfer calcium into your bones, chia supports bone health too!

GROW YOUR OWN

Try sprinkling chia seeds on the ground and covering them with a thin layer of soil. Water them gently and you will see how easily and willingly the chia grows.

The plant produces beautiful purple flowers and, once the flower heads dry out, you will have your own chia seeds ready to use in the kitchen or to sow once again in the garden.

HOW WE USE CHIA

The taste of chia is very mild and pleasant and easily combines with other foods without changing the taste dramatically. Chia can be added to recipes to provide more bulk and nutritional density. The most common way to eat chia is to first soak the seeds. They rapidly absorb lots of liquid—between nine and twelve times their volume in under ten minutes.

Chia can be used as a gel or in its whole-seed form. Enjoy it as a porridge, add it to smoothies, mix it into soups, sauces, energy bars, crackers, or desserts.

YOU CAN FEED CHIA SEEDS TO YOUR PETS TOO! THEY THRIVE ON IT. BERYN FEEDS CHIA SEEDS TO HER HORSES. THE GOOD OILS KEEP THEM HEALTHY AND MAKE THEIR COATS SHINY AND LAVISH. IT DOES THE SAME FOR OUR HAIR.

ONCE YOU HAVE A WHOLE LOT OF CHIA GROWING TALL AND HEALTHY, TAKE A PEEK UNDERNEATH TO SEE IF YOU CAN SPOT THE SHY AND ELUSIVE CHIA MONSTER.

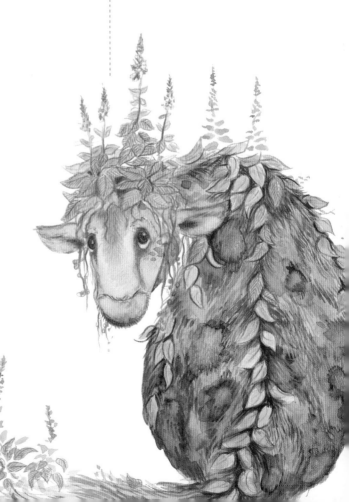

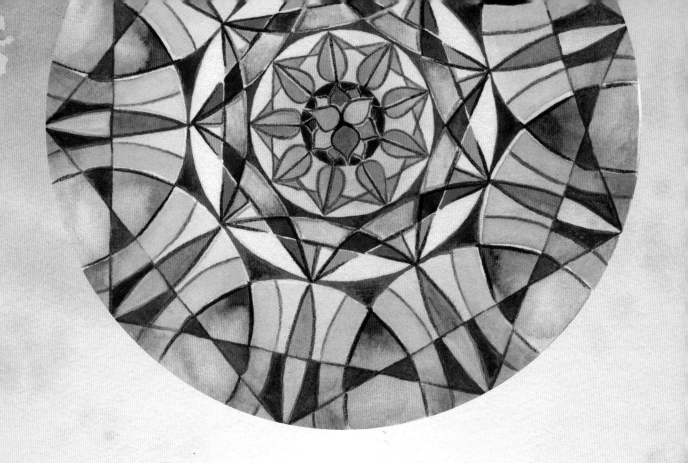

CHIA RECIPES

CHIA PORRIDGE * FRUIT SALAD AND CHIA WITH NUT MILK

WARM CHIA OAT PORRIDGE * CHIA OMEGA SUPER-MILK * CHOC OMEGA SUPER-MILK

CHIA OMEGA CREAM * CHIA CAULIFLOWER SOUP * CHIA, TOMATO, AND ONION CRACKERS

CHIA CURRY * RUNNER`S BAR

CHIA PORRIDGE

Chia seeds are rich in omega-3s, making this a perfect brain-food breakfast.

> 3 T chia seeds
> water

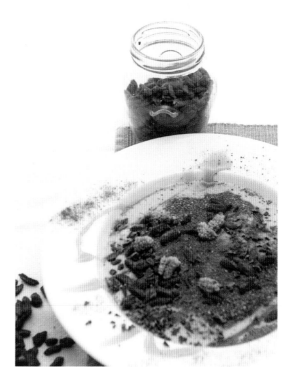

Cover the chia seeds in water and allow them to soak up the water for five minutes. From here, you are free to dress your chia porridge in any number of ways.

The following are some of our favorite variations.

Chia porridge with mulberry milk or almond milk, cinnamon, and honey

> mulberry milk (see page 81) or almond milk (see page 209)
> ½ t ground cinnamon
> 1 t honey (or to taste)
> 10 white mulberries

Take your soaked chia seeds and cover with mulberry milk. Add cinnamon and honey, and top with white mulberries.

Supreme superfood chia porridge

> lucuma powder
> mesquite powder
> maca powder
> cacao powder
> cacao nibs
> goji berries
> honey

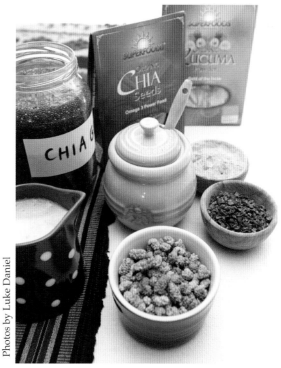

Take your soaked chia seeds and add any of the above ingredients in desired quantities. Add extra water and stir together.

Time-saving tip: Pre-prepare your chia gel. Chia gel keeps well in the fridge for up to a week. Take 1 C chia and cover with 4 C water. Allow it to soak and become a gel. Store in a 1-qt glass jar in the fridge and use by the spoonful as required.

Photos by Luke Daniel

Chia Recipes   65

FRUIT SALAD AND CHIA WITH NUT MILK

a selection of seasonal fruit: pawpaw, banana, strawberries, blueberries, gooseberries, passion fruit
a generous dollop of chia gel
nut milk of your choice
a selection of superfoods: cacao nibs, goji berries, raw honey, hemp seeds, bee pollen

Every so often, we still love to start the day off with a fruit salad. We super-zoop it up with some superfoods, including of course a generous dollop of chia gel, which we call chia glupe!

Dice 2–3 different types of seasonal fresh fruit into a bowl. Add a generous portion of chia gel. Pour over nut milk. Top with your favorite superfoods.

WARM CHIA OAT PORRIDGE

Serves 2

1 C hot water
½ C raw oats
4 T chia seeds
2 T coconut oil
2 T cacao butter
2 T goji berries
2 T lucuma powder
2 T hemp seeds
2 T cacao nibs
2 T honey
2 T cacao powder (optional)

This is a fantastic winter warming breakfast recipe.

Cover the oats with hot water and allow to stand for two minutes to soak and soften. Add the rest of the ingredients and stir. Add more water if too thick.

CHIA OMEGA SUPER-MILK

3 C water
¼ C hemp seeds
⅛ C chia seeds
¼ C lucuma powder
1–2 T honey (depending on how sweet you prefer)
½ t vanilla seeds

Hemp and chia seeds combined give you a fantastic omega super-milk. With lucuma and honey for extra flavor, this is a delicious no-nut milk that can be used as a base for all types of smoothies.

Blend together and allow to stand for 1–2 minutes to thicken.

CHOC OMEGA SUPER-MILK

Take the chia omega super-milk recipe. Blend in ¼ C cacao powder.

CHIA OMEGA CREAM

The chia omega super-milk recipe is such a versatile recipe. To make a thick cream version, simply use 1 C water instead of 3 C.

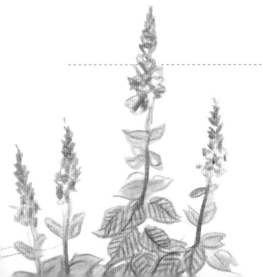

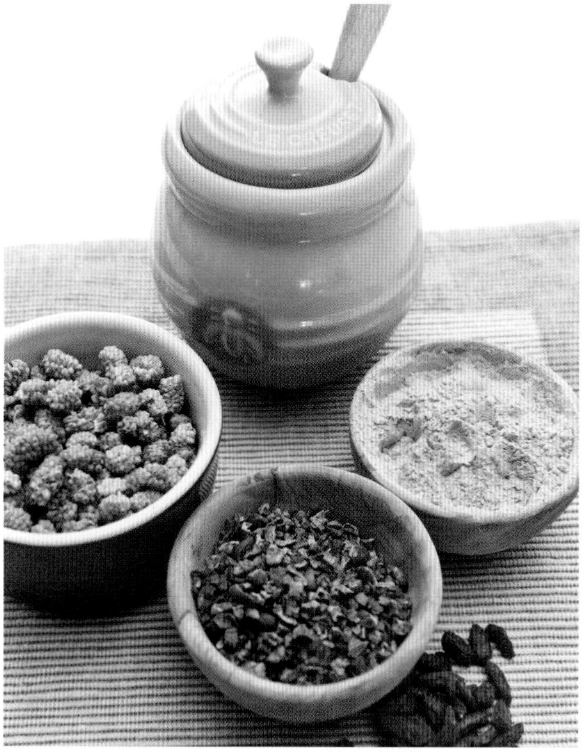

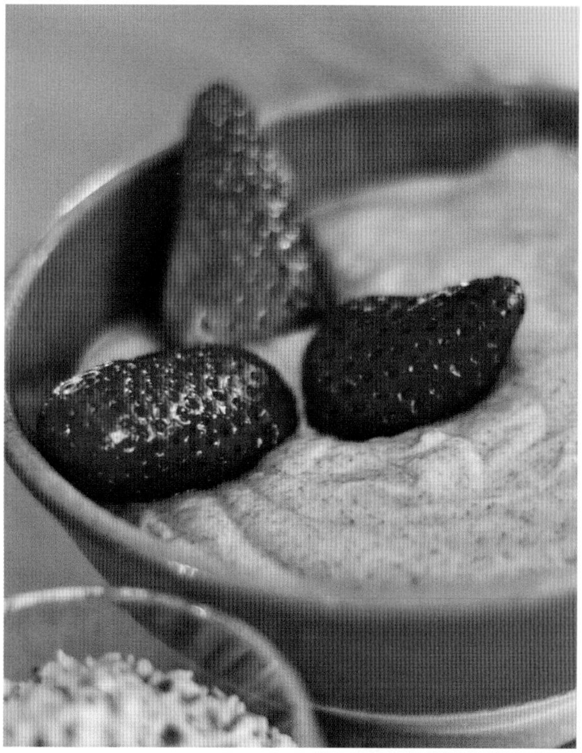

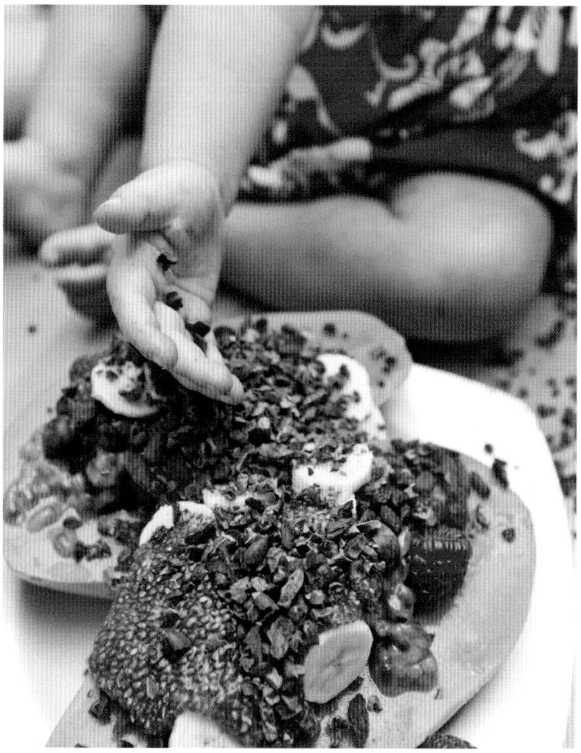

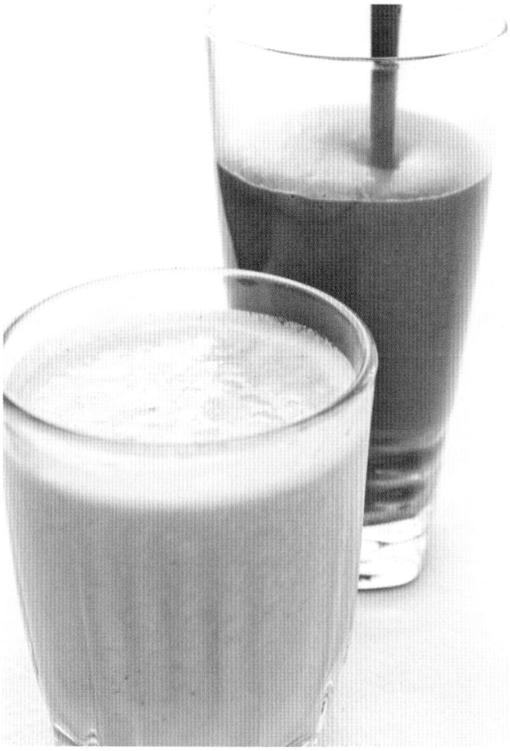

Photos by Luke Daniel

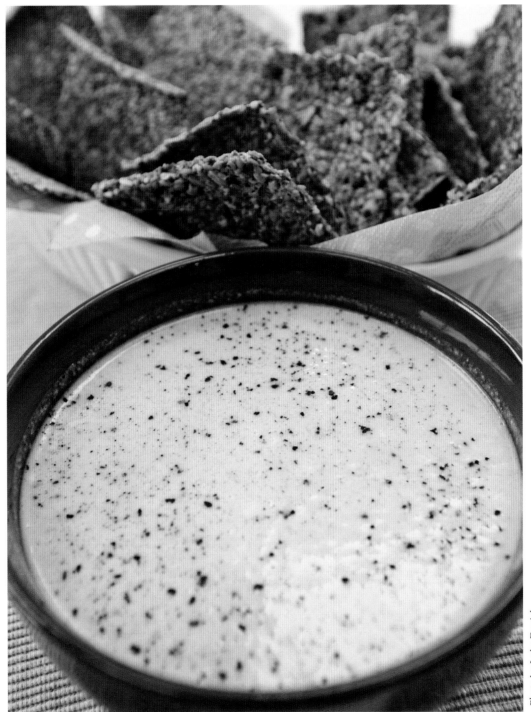

CHIA AND CAULIFLOWER SOUP

The chia seeds in this recipe help to thicken the soup.

Blend the ingredients, preferably in a high-speed blender. Serve with chia crackers (see below).

Makes 2 qt

> *1 qt hot water*
> *½ cauliflower (covered in warm water to soften)*
> *½ avocado*
> *¼ C chia seeds*
> *¼ C cashews or macadamias*
> *¼ onion*
> *1 garlic clove*
> *1 T nutritional yeast*
> *1 T hemp oil*
> *2 t miso*
> *1 t salt*
> *½ t black pepper (optional)*

CHIA, TOMATO, AND ONION CRACKERS

Soak the flax and chia in the water for ten minutes. In a food processor or blender, blend up the tomatoes, onion, and salt. Add the soaked flax and chia and pulse through. Spread out the mixture onto teflex dehydrator sheets. I like to sprinkle extra salt over the wet mixture and score them into the desired shapes at this point, so that they break cleanly later. Dehydrate for 12–14 hours. After 1–2 hours of drying time you can remove the teflex sheet, after which the crackers will dry more swiftly. I use an Excalibur dehydrator and the mixture covers two trays (12 x 12 in), which amounts to approximately 18 crackers.

Makes 18 crackers

> *1 C golden flaxseeds*
> *½ C chia seeds*
> *2 C water*
> *4 large tomatoes*
> *½ onion*
> *1 t salt*

Mega-seed version

When you are adding the soaked flax and chia to the blended tomato and onion, simply add the following dry ingredients:

> *½ C hemp seeds*
> *½ C pumpkin seeds*
> *½ C sunflower seeds*

Continue as above.

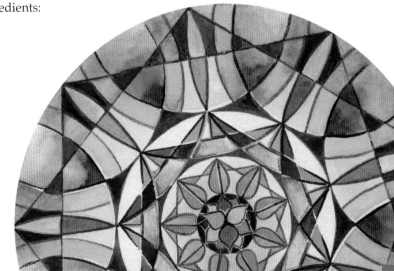

Serves 4

For the sauce:

> 2¼ lb cherry tomatoes
> ½ C red onion, chopped
> ¼ C light oil, such as maca-
> damia nut or sunflower seed
> ¼ C honey
> 3 T tamari
> 2 T fresh ginger, minced
> 2 t curry powder, mild
> 2 t garam masala
> 1 t kelp powder
> ½ t turmeric powder
> 2 garlic cloves
> 1 t salt
> chili for extra heat (optional)

Pulse in:

> 1¾ C (400 g) cherry tomatoes
> ¼ C (50 g) fresh coriander
> ⅔ C chia seeds

Stir in:

> ¾ C (150 g) peas
> ¾ C (150 g) baby spinach

CHIA CURRY

This recipe has been contributed from *Easy Living Food* by Natalie Reid and Noel Marten and is a fantastic savory chia dish. It is called *Tamaatar chia kadhi.*

Blend all the sauce ingredients until smooth and warm for about one minute. Next, put the pulse ingredients into the blender and pulse just once or twice to chop and mix.

Let this stand for ten minutes for the chia to work its magic. Put the peas and spinach into a pot and mix in the sauce. Warm everything on low heat and serve with veggie "rice" (see page 163, parsnip rice).

Makes 20 bars

> ¾ C chia seeds
> ¼ C lucuma powder
> ¼ C cacao powder
> 3 T hemp powder
> 2 T mesquite powder
> 2 T maca
> 2 T wheatgrass powder
> 2 T honey
> 1 T ashwagandha
> 1 T spirulina powder
> 1 T foti
> ¼ t Himalayan rock salt

For the date jam:

> 1½ C dates, soaked
> 2 C water

RUNNER`S BAR

Peter's brother, Werner, is a superfoods athlete. He recently took up trail running and has been doing phenomenally well! This is his chia runner's bar recipe that he uses to power up for training and racing.

In a power blender or seed grinder, grind the chia seeds into a fine powder.

Combine with all the other superfoods in a bowl. In a separate bowl, blend the dates and water into a date paste, and pour over the dry mixture. Work through into a paste.

As a nice finishing touch, place some goji berries on top.

Dehydrate for 12–16 hours and store in the fridge.

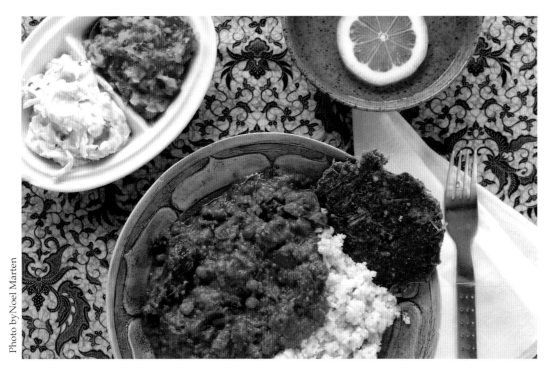

Photo by Noel Marten

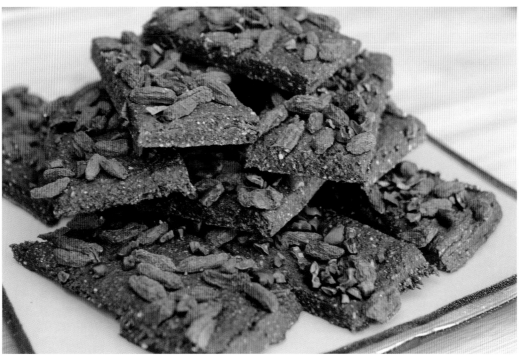

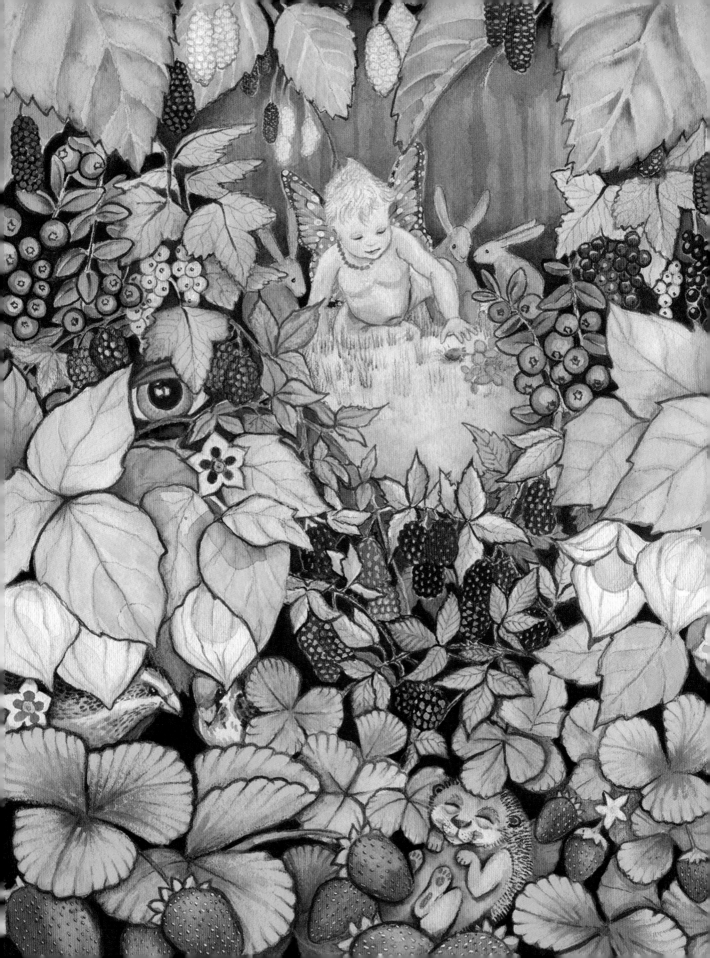

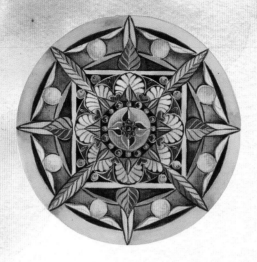

BERRIES
BEAUTIFUL BOUNTY

LONGEVITY ANTIOXIDANTS • WEIGHT LOSS NUTRIENT DENSITY
LOWERING BLOOD PRESSURE • ANTICARCINOGENIC • CARDIOVASCULAR HEALTH
COMBATING URINARY TRACT INFECTIONS • COGNITIVE BENEFITS
BALANCING BLOOD SUGAR

Down in the garden in a brambly hedgerow,
Or in the forest, is where berries grow.
Sometimes on bushes, on vines or on trees
It's possible to find delicious treats such as these
In a rainbow of colors, from red to blue-black
Little nutrition bombs, nature's sweet snack.
A bountiful harvest all foraged by you,
Can make you feel connected to Nature too
It reminds you that you're supported in the earth's embrace
That you're never alone while you're in this place
You're surrounded by love, you are watched, and you're guided
You can trust that in life all you need is provided.

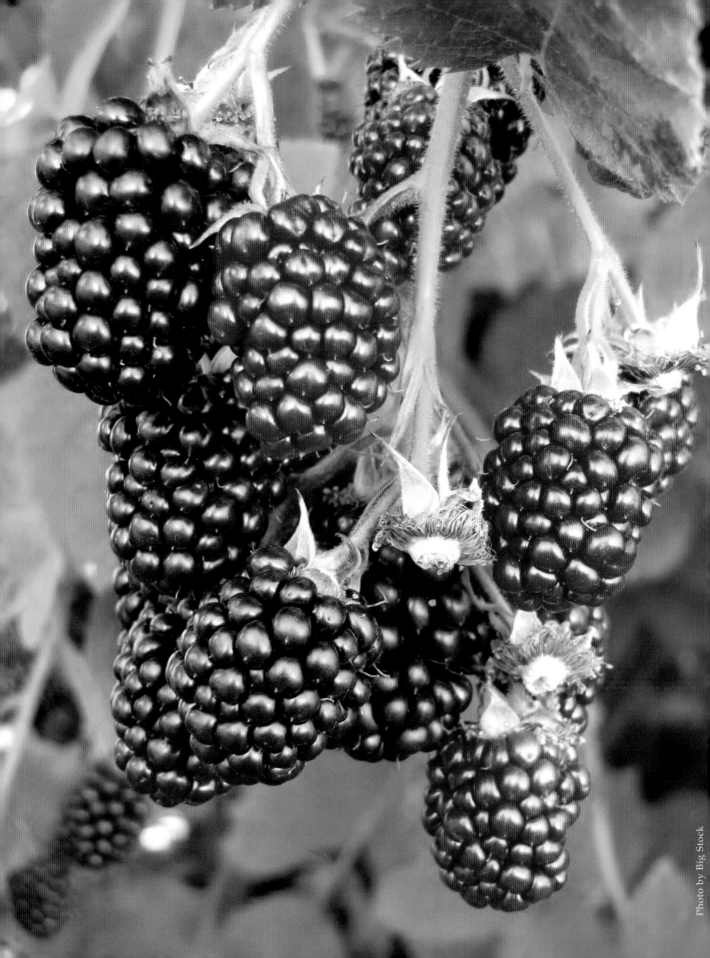

ANCIENT, REVERED SUPERFOOD

Berries are one of the most perfect foods for people to regularly eat. Our ancestors foraged for them for thousands of years. They grow easily like weeds, birds spread their seeds, and we get the resulting bright-colored, tasty, and nutrient-dense gifts of nature.

Raspberries, blueberries, blackberries, cranberries, and strawberries are just a few of your choices. Berries are a vital part of our nutrition, mainly because of the phytochemicals they contain. Phytochemicals protect your cells from damage—scientists are finding that berries have some of the highest antioxidant levels of any fruit. When it comes to fruit, it's hard to beat the nutrient profile of berries. Berries are powerful superfoods rich in fiber, vitamins, minerals, antioxidants, and phytochemicals, which may help prevent (and, in some cases, reverse) the effects of aging, cardiovascular disease, arthritis, diabetes, high blood pressure, and certain types of cancer. According to the American Institute for Cancer Research, many cancer-fighting nutrients can be found in all types of berries.

In botanical language, a berry is a simple fruit having seeds and pulp produced from a single ovary. This group includes foods that you wouldn't expect: avocado, banana, grape, pumpkin, and watermelon! This is obviously not what we think of when looking for berries—we are usually thinking of forest berries. Forest berries are available fresh during summer and include raspberries, blueberries, blackberries, gooseberries, and strawberries, to name but a few. Then there are the lesser-known wild berries and region-specific superberries. We will describe some of them in this chapter.

A. BLUEBERRIES WON'T RIPEN ONCE THEY'VE BEEN PICKED

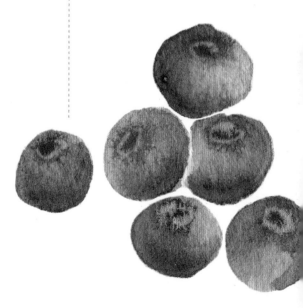

Berries   75

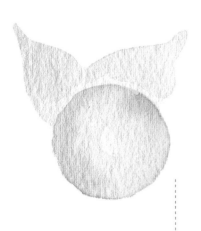

ORGANIC BERRIES

Unfortunately, commercially grown berries are often on the "dirty dozen" list of foods tested to be most highly contaminated with pesticide and herbicide residues. Strawberries are almost always near the top of the list. These are highly toxic chemicals that have no place on earth, let alone on the food we eat or in our bodies. Contact your berry supplier to ask if they test for residues. If organic berries are available, pick or buy as many as you can, feast on as many as you can eat (or afford), and freeze the rest! Plant berry bushes in your garden: grow your own superfoods and produce your own beautiful summer bounty.

SUGGESTION: GO FORAGING IN BERRY SEASON AND FREEZE THE EXCESS TO USE THROUGHOUT THE REST OF THE YEAR!

Raspberries

Slightly tart and juicy, raspberries are rich in ellagic acid, which provides the majority of the berry's antioxidants and antimicrobial anthocyanins, which give raspberries their deep, red color. They are also a great source of vitamins and minerals such as riboflavin, niacin, folate, magnesium, potassium, copper, manganese, and vitamin C.

Blueberries

Blueberries are small and famous. They are known for their anti-inflammatory and antibacterial properties and are among the most powerful sources of antioxidants as well as B vitamins, fiber, and vitamins C, E, and K. The cancer-fighting phytochemicals found specifically in blueberries include anthocyanins and resveratrol.

Blackberries

These are berries widely found growing wild as brambles. In the wild they are small and tart. Their cultivated cousins are plump, dark, and juicy, and are another delicious source of antioxidant anthocyanin pigments and ellagic acids, as well as vitamins C and E, fiber, and the phytochemical lycopene, which protects eyesight.

Strawberries

It's easy to see why strawberries are one of the most popular berries. Fragrant, sweet, and juicy, strawberries taste as good as they are for you! This rich source of vitamin C, folate, fiber, and B vitamins also contains phytonutrients and antioxidants, such as phenols. These elements give strawberries heart-protecting, anti-inflammatory, and anticarcinogenic properties. Strawberries are

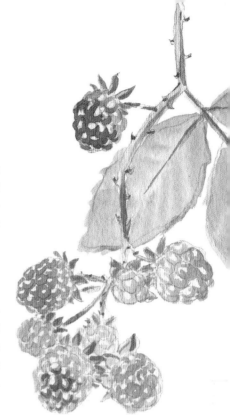

a good source of antioxidants and folic acid and an excellent source of vitamin C, which has been shown to decrease the risk of esophageal cancer. One cup of strawberries provides 100% of your daily recommended vitamin C. As beautiful as they look, they often hide a dark secret: they are likely covered with toxic herbicides if not certified organic.

Mulberries

Highly valued in the Roman Empire since ancient times, these sweet and nutritious fruits are high in vitamin C, iron, calcium, and protein, and are a good source of colon-supporting dietary fiber. In Chinese medicine, mulberries are classified as a blood tonic. Mulberries are a source of resveratrol, which blocks the action of cancer-causing agents, inhibiting tumor growth and development. They also contain anthocyanins, which guard against cardiovascular disease.

Incan berries or Cape gooseberries

Incan berries originate from Peru and Brazil. They were brought to England in 1774 and then to South Africa, specifically the Cape, in the early 1800s as an easy-to-grow crop, high in vitamin C, to supply passing ships on their long voyages to the East. Incan berries are packed with antioxidants, minerals, and vitamins, helping to stabilize blood sugar levels. They grow like weeds in our garden and are very easy to propagate from the seeds in the berries.

Acai berry

Acai is the Brazilian palm berry. Acai contains some of the highest antioxidant capacity of any food. The acai berry became very popular in large Brazilian cities in the late 1980s, and has since become popular worldwide. Acai berry contains amino acids, protein, and various vitamins, including vitamins A, B1, B2, B3, C, E, and K. It contains very high amounts of niacin and vitamin B6. Acai berries also contain a variety of minerals, including magnesium, zinc, calcium, copper, and potassium. Acai berry contains many polyphenolic anthocyanin compounds such as resveratrol, cyanidin-3-galactoside, ferulic acid, delphinidin, and petunidin, as well as astringent pro-anthocyanidin tannins such as epicatechin, protocatechuic acid, and ellagic acid. Scientific studies suggest that these compounds have anti-aging, anti-inflammatory, and anticarcinogenic functions by virtue of the way they fight free radicals. In addition, tannins are known to have anti-infective, anti-inflammatory, and anti-hemorrhagic properties.

Cranberries

These tart and tangy berries are sources of polyphenols, antioxidants that may benefit the cardiovascular system and immune system and act as anticarcinogenic agents. They also contain tannins, with anti-clotting properties. Besides being a rich source of antioxidants, cranberries also boast fiber, vitamins A and C, potassium, and more. Cranberries are rarely eaten fresh since they are so sour. Instead, cranberries are often dried and sweetened with refined sugar, which strips minerals from the body.

Bilberries

The bilberrry has one of the highest levels of anthocyanin of all berries. It is a forest fruit native to Europe. In Europe it is often referred to generically as "blueberry," but there are significant differences between the bilberry and the typical North American blueberry. The blueberry has a high concentration of anthocyanins in the outer skin, but has greenish flesh. The bilberry has a blue skin and reddish flesh, indicating a higher concentration of anthocyanins throughout the berry.

Currants

The currant, especially the black currant, is a high-antioxidant berry. The currant has been enjoyed for generations in Europe. The wonderful flavor cassis is derived from the black currant, and is one of the most popular berry flavors in Europe.

Elderberries

The elderberry is very high in anthocyanins, antioxidants, and polyphenolics in general.

Maquis berries

The maquis berry, from Chile, is one of the newest entrants to the superfruit category. It has a very high anthocyanin and total phenolic content, like acai and bilberry.

Rose hips

Rose hips are only now being recognized as a superfruit. Rose hips are high in vitamin C, lycopene, antioxidant flavonoids, and other nutritional compounds.

Sea buckthorn

Sea buckthorn is a yellowish berry with very high levels of carotenoids, betacarotene, and related compounds.

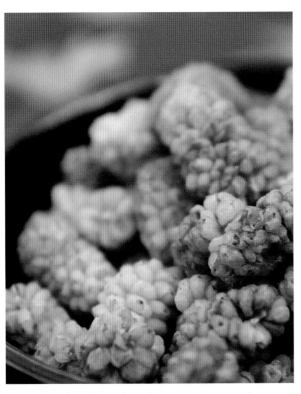
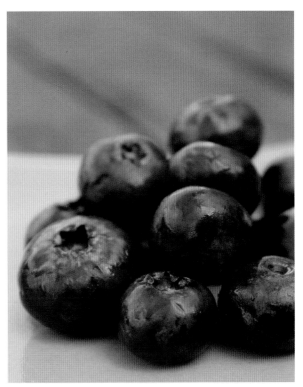
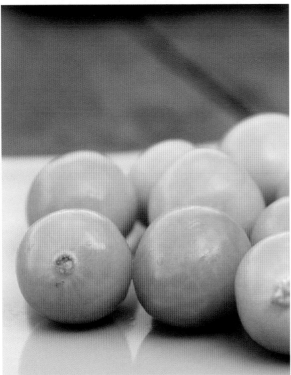
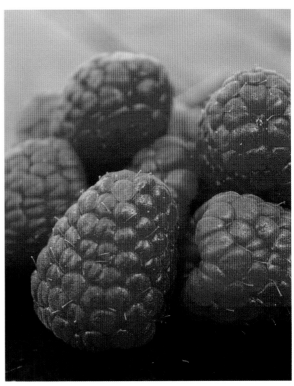

THE MAGIC OF BERRIES

- LONGEVITY ANTIOXIDANTS
- WEIGHT LOSS NUTRIENT DENSITY
- LOWERING BLOOD PRESSURE
- ANTICARCINOGENIC
- CARDIOVASCULAR HEALTH
- COMBATING URINARY TRACT INFECTIONS
- COGNITIVE BENEFITS
- BALANCING BLOOD SUGAR

Longevity antioxidants

Berries are packed with the bright pigments of antioxidants, protecting cells from stress and allowing them to function optimally. Virtually every body system studied shows improvement when antioxidant-rich berries are consumed.

STRAWBERRIES ARE THE ONLY FRUIT THAT GROWS SEEDS ON THE OUTSIDE, WITH OVER 200 SEEDS ON EVERY BERRY.

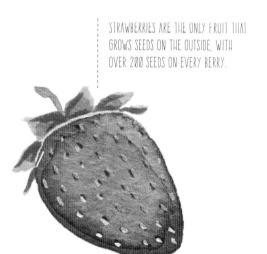

Weight loss nutrient density

Berries are ideal as a weight-loss food. They're sweet and delicious without lots of calories or fat, and rich in nutrients such as pectin, a soluble fiber that promotes a feeling of fullness.

Lowering blood pressure

Antioxidants fight the systemic inflammation that comes with having high blood pressure. The intake of berries can significantly reduce both systolic and diastolic blood pressures. This is why so many doctors recommend eating a lot of fruit and vegetables if you have high blood pressure.

Anticarcinogenic properties

While almost exclusively coming in the form of laboratory studies on human cells, an increasing percentage of berry research is being focused on anticarcinogenic benefits. It seems as though the powerful phytonutrient ellagic acid in berries is responsible for their anticarcinogenic effect. This compound is located in berry seeds, and various studies have demonstrated that people who consume foods high in ellagic acid are three times less likely to develop cancer.

Cardiovascular health

The antioxidant defenses provided by berries have been especially well documented with respect to the cardiovascular system. It's the many different pathways for cardio support that are so striking in berry research. In repeated studies of blood composition, blueberry intake has been shown to improve blood fat balances, including reduction in total cholesterol, raising of HDL cholesterol, and lowering of triglycerides. It has also been shown that berry intake provides protection for the cells lining the

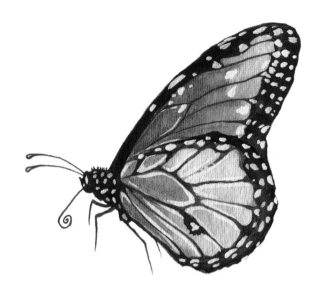

blood vessel walls. Connected with this antioxidant protection of blood vessel structures and blood fats is an improved overall antioxidant capacity in the blood itself. Increased activity of an enzyme called nitric oxide synthase, endogenous NOS or eNOS, is usually associated with better balance in cardiovascular function. Recent studies have shown that daily blueberry intake can result in increased eNOS activity, which is viewed as helping to explain some of the unique health benefits of blueberries for the cardiovascular system. Berries are also rich in folate, which supports the cardiovascular system by decreasing inflammatory homocysteine levels.

Combating urinary tract infections

Researchers have found that cranberry juice in particular could prevent the formation of urinary tract infections. Cranberries contain a substance that prevents infection-causing bacteria from sticking to the walls of the urinary tract.

Cognitive benefits

Research studies on berry intake suggest that a large part of the cognitive benefit is most likely due to blueberries' vast array of antioxidant nutrients protecting nerve cells from oxygen damage. Nerve cells have a naturally high risk of oxygen damage and they require special antioxidant protection at all times in life. By lowering the risk of oxidative stress in our nerve cells, blueberries help us maintain smoothly working nerve cells and healthy cognitive function.

Balancing blood sugar

Berries are ideal for a diabetic diet. They're sweet, delicious, and low on the glycemic index. Fresh strawberries, blueberries, blackberries, and rasp-

berries all have scores below 40. They also provide a very good amount of fiber, which, together with their low GI, is helpful in blood sugar regulation.

HOW WE USE BERRIES

If fresh berries were available all year, they would be a major part of our diet. They are so nourishing, gentle, and supportive, yet nutrient-rich, that they can and should be eaten by the bucket load when in season. Picking berries in the wild or from your own bushes is a rewarding and magical activity. Homegrown berries always taste so much more intense. Of course, berries can and should be eaten just as they are. We also use them in smoothies, to make delicious berry nut-milkshakes, ice creams, raw cakes, and more!

WARNINGS

Beware of wild harvesting; not all berries are edible, and many berries are toxic and can even be fatal.

BERRY RECIPES

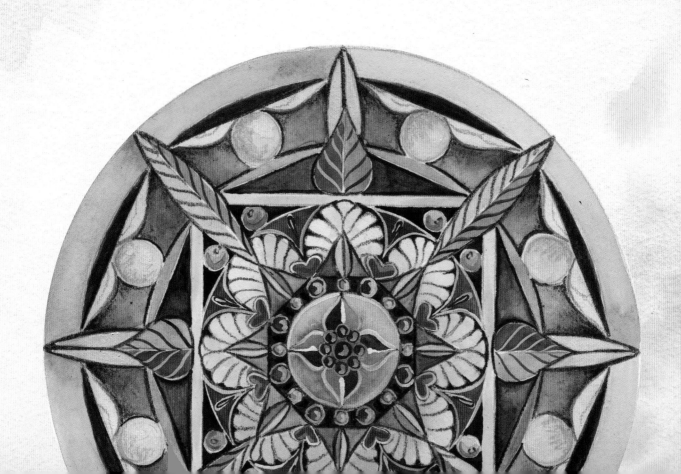

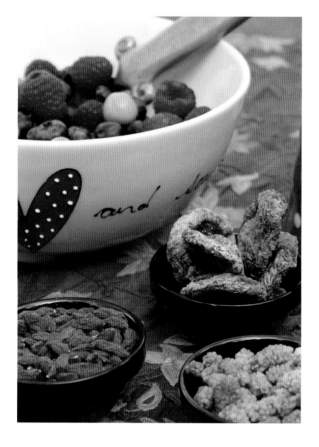

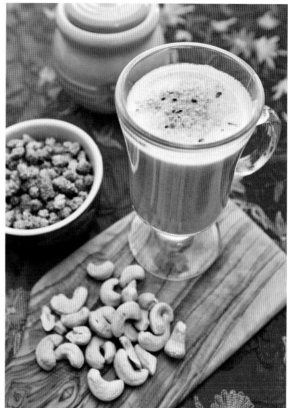

BERRY BREAKFAST

In summertime indulge in the abundance of berries. Create a fruit salad of the best fresh berries you can find, such as strawberries, raspberries, blueberries, blackberries, and gooseberries. Top with dried mulberries, goji berries, and figs (fresh or dried).

Tip: We like to add 2 T chia gel and some chia omega milk or chia omega cream (see page 64) and sprinkle with cacao nibs. Or if we're feeling very decadent, chocolate sauce on berries for breakfast is our version of "breakfast like a king."

WARM MULBERRY MILK

This mulberry milk is delicious warm on a cold day. You can also use this sweet warm milk as a base for hot chocolate or use it cold as a base for scrumptious smoothies.

> 2 C hot or cold water
> ¼ C dried white mulberries
> ¼ C cashews
> 1 T hemp seeds
> 1 T honey

Blend ingredients together and enjoy!

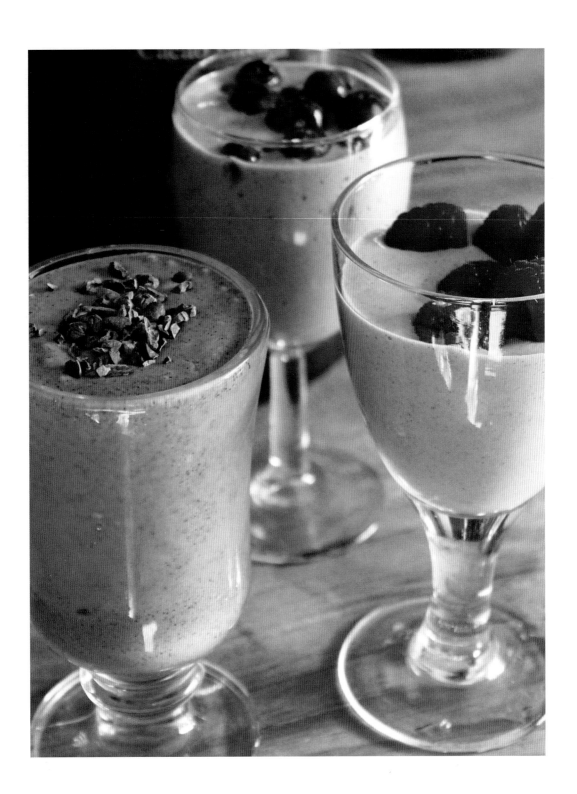

OTHER BERRY MILKS

2 C hemp milk (see page 131), almond milk (see page 209),
   or mulberry milk (see page 81)
1 C fresh or frozen berries
1 T honey (for extra sweetness)

Blend and enjoy.

LEXI'S MIXED BERRY DELIGHT

This is a scrumptious contribution from our illustrator, Alexis. Her favorite time is when black mulberries and blackberries are fruiting—it turns this drink deep burgundy! "Drinking this feels like a blood transfusion, with the deep purple-red color and the yummy choc chips."

Blend the Brazil nuts, water, honey, and vanilla seeds. Add the berries and process until smooth. Add a handful of cacao nibs and process lightly to disperse the "choc chips." Pour into a tall glass and sip, or eat with a spoon! Divine on a hot day!

Makes 3 C

½ C frozen blackberries or
   mulberries
½ C frozen blueberries (or
   combination of berries of
   your choice)
½ C water
¼ C Brazil nuts
1 T honey (or sweeten to taste)
seeds of 1 vanilla pod
a handful of cacao nibs

BERRY BLISS SMOOTHIE

Blend everything in a blender. Pour into glasses.

Makes 2 C

1 C fresh strawberries,
   raspberries, blackberries, or
   blueberries
1 large banana
1 C hemp milk (see page 131)
1 T honey
1 T coconut oil
¼ t vanilla extract or seeds
   of 1 vanilla pod
½ t cinnamon
pinch of Himalayan rock salt

For red, orange, and yellow:

raspberries
nasturtium flowers
gooseberries

For green:

wild rocket
finely sliced spinach
thinly sliced avocado
parsley

For blue, indigo, and violet:

blackberries and blueberries
borage flowers
and any other wild edible
*   flowers*

RAINBOW SALAD

Combine these ingredients in desired quantities as available for the most colorful salad imaginable.

Serve with raspberry dressing (see below).

Makes 1 C

½ C raspberries
½ C olive oil
juice of 1 lemon
1 T honey
⅛ C Rosendal vinegar
¼ t salt

RASPBERRY DRESSING

Blend all ingredients together and serve with a salad.

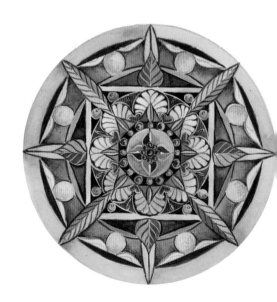

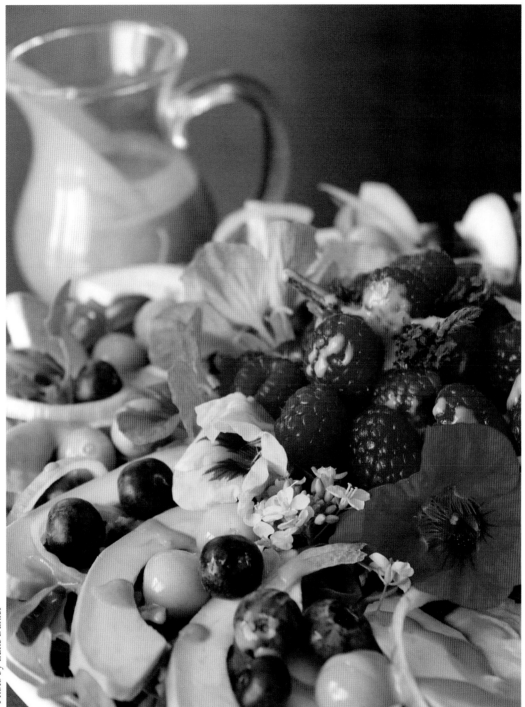

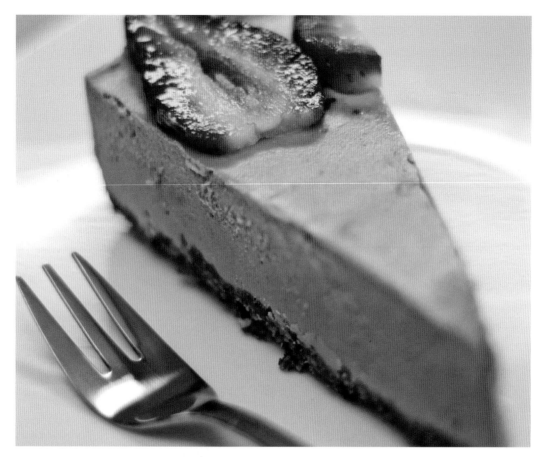

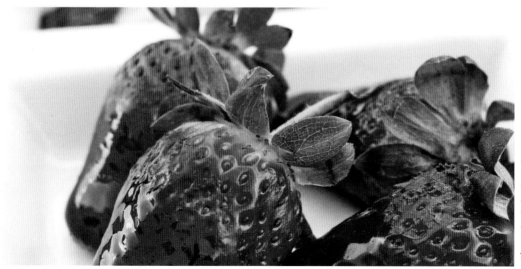

CHOC-BERRY CHEESECAKE

You can make a variety of different color cakes using this simple recipe. At our DVD launch, we served a pink (strawberry) version, a yellow (mango topped with gooseberries) version, a green (spirulina) version (see page 99), and a purple (blueberry) version. It was a feast for the eyes and the tummies.

Put all the base ingredients into a food processor and blend until finely chopped. Press into the base of a springform cake tin, puncture holes in the base using a fork, and put it into the fridge while you make the filling.

Blend all the ingredients for the filling together in a power blender until smooth. Make a double batch if you want a really tall cake. Pour the filling over the base. Decorate with berries of choice. Refrigerate overnight or place in the freezer to set. The coconut oil in the recipe helps the cake to set once you put it in the fridge or freezer.

Serves 10–12

For the chocolate base:

> *2 C pecans*
> *¼ C cacao powder*
> *¼ C mesquite powder*
> *2 T honey*
> *2 T coconut oil*
> *¼ t Himalayan salt*

For the filling:

> *1 C cashew nuts, soaked*
> *1 C macadamias, soaked*
> *1 C coconut oil*
> *¾ C honey*
> *¼ C lemon juice*
> *1 T vanilla extract*
> *3 C fresh strawberries or raspberries—for a pink cake*
> *3 C blueberries or blackberries—for a purple cake*
> *2 C mangoes and gooseberries—for a yellow cake*

For the topping:

> *berries of your choice*

CHOC-DIPPED FRUIT

This is the easiest way to serve a dessert that is decadent and delicious.

Chill your strawberries in the freezer while you make a batch of chocolate sauce. Dip them in chocolate and set them in the fridge.

strawberries
chocolate sauce (see page 229)

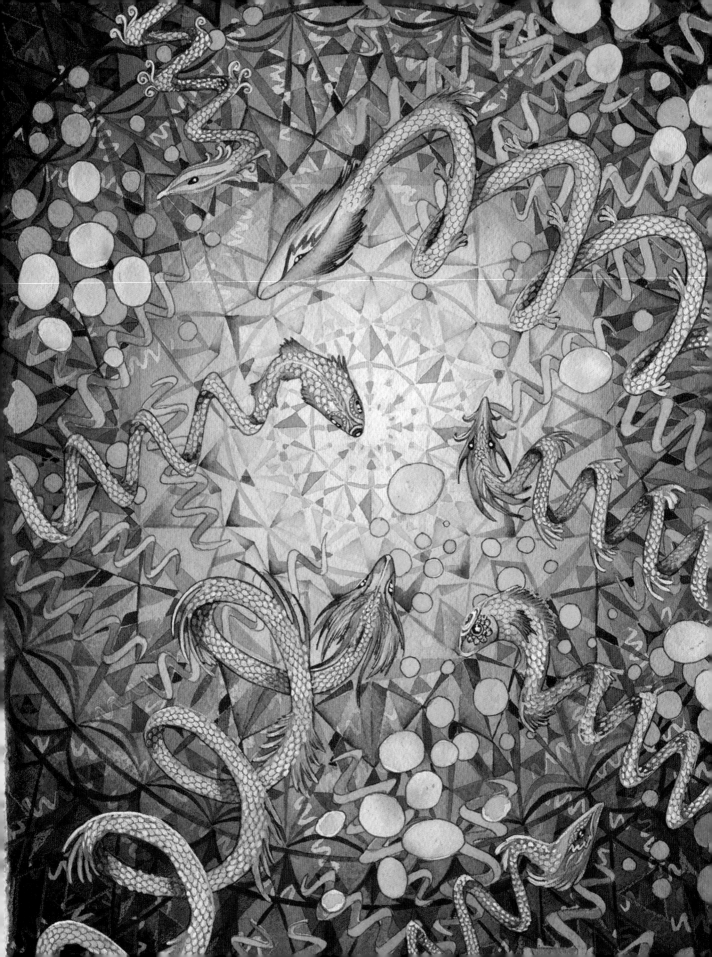

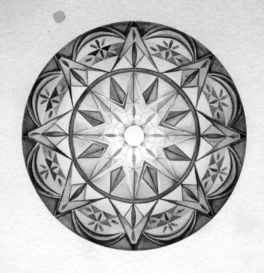

BLUE-GREEN ALGAE
PRIMORDIAL ORIGINAL FOOD

—∞—∞—∞—∞—∞—∞—∞—∞—∞—

PROTEIN POWER * BOOSTS IMMUNE FUNCTION

ENERGY BOOSTING * CLEANSING CHLOROPHYLL

STRESS RELIEF AND NATURAL ANTIDEPRESSANT * METAL DETOXING

BLOOD BUILDING * LONGEVITY * WEIGHT LOSS * GLA SUPER OIL

—∞—∞—∞—∞—∞—∞—∞—∞—∞—

A swirling spectrum, primordial soup,
The ancestors of plant life, a spiraling loop.
Since the sun shone young and bright in the ancient earth's sky,
Algae have flourished and nourished, both deep and high.
Amazing Algae Aqua Dragons, so rich in nutrition
Can offer food and fuel: an abundant vision.
Life's building blocks are all herein contained,
In a dance with sun's rays we can all be sustained.
And, what's more, do you know what else they do?
They create breathable air, for me and for you.
Three quarters of all earth's oxygen's from the sea,
Produced by algae, in service of earth, you, and me!

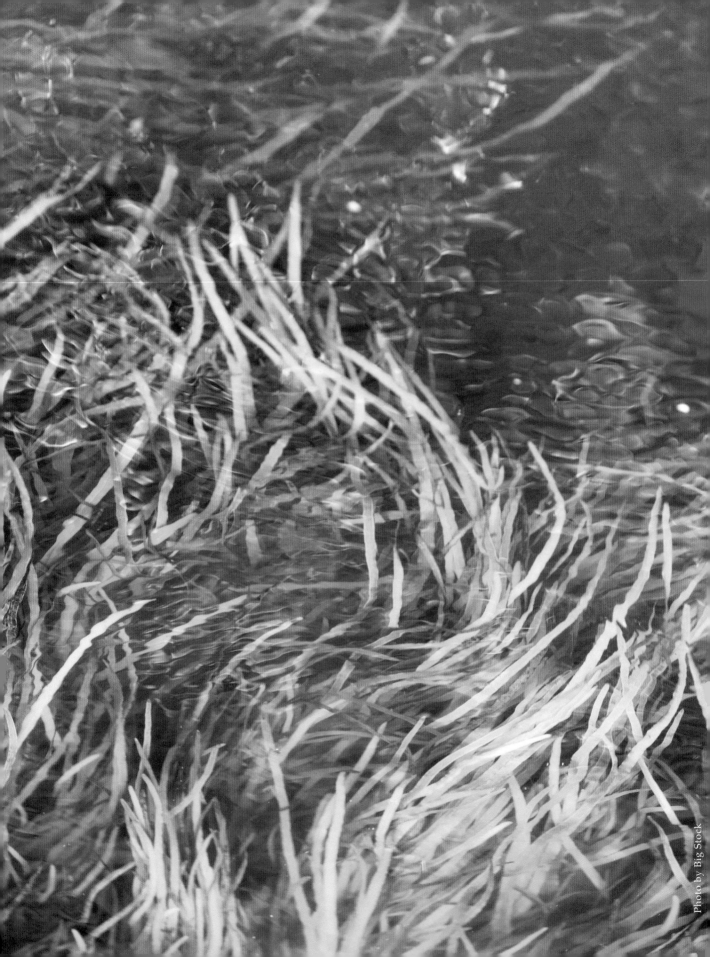

ANCIENT, REVERED SUPERFOOD

People have understood the importance of blue-green algae as a food source for at least four thousand years; Chinese herbalists have been using it to treat diseases for thousands of years. The Mayans and Aztecs regularly ate freshly harvested algae. The tribes living near Lake Chad in the African Sahara are still making and eating algae cakes.

Blue-green algae are the primordial food and have been around for 3.5 billion years. They are microscopic plants that grow in freshwater. They contain the highest nutrient values and use up the least amount of the planet's resources. Collectively, algae supply 90% of the world's oxygen and potentially 80% of its food. Blue-green algae are also at the bottom of the food chain, meaning lower concentrations of toxins, biocides, and environmental pollutants. Looking at the nutrients algae provide, a well-informed nutritionist can only stand in awe: these are many of the nutrients needed by every human body, in near-perfect ratios! It's almost as if Mother Nature herself reached out from the waters and said, "Here is the perfect food for all human beings" and gave us micro-algae. They're that impressive. There are three main types of algae commonly consumed today, namely AFA blue-green algae, spirulina, and chlorella.

AFA blue-green algae

AFA is a particular type of wild blue-green algae, found abundantly in Klamath Lake in Oregon. It contains virtually every nutrient, with a 60% protein content and a more complete amino acid profile than beef or soy beans. AFA contains brain-specific phytochemicals, antioxidants, minerals, vitamins, and enzymes. It is one of the richest food sources of betacarotene, B vitamins, and chlorophyll. It has been shown to improve brain function and memory, strengthen the immune system, and help fight viruses, colds, and flu.

Spirulina

Spirulina is a cultivated blue-green algae that occurs naturally in the highly alkaline volcanic lakes of Africa and Mexico. It has been consumed for thousands of years by indigenous peoples. Spirulina gets its name from its spiral DNA-like shape when seen through a microscope. Spirulina contains a phenomenal combination of protein, vitamins, minerals, EFAs, phytonutrients, RNA, DNA, and antioxidants. Studies have shown that spirulina can help control blood sugar levels and cravings, thus making it a key food for diabetics, and can be used to assist in weight loss and as a general nutritional supplement.

Chlorella

Chlorella is a fresh-water algae and, like its other algae cousins, contains a complete protein profile, all the B vitamins, vitamins C and E, and many minerals. It is amazing for the immune system and for reducing cholesterol and preventing the hardening of arteries. It is particularly powerful as a detoxing agent, assisting the body to release heavy metals such as mercury.

Toxic algae

Many species of algae contain dangerous toxins, including neurotoxins. The three species mentioned here have been safely used as food sources for thousands of years as well as intensely tested for toxicity by scientists for decades. They have been found to be completely safe. As with other plants, quality is key, so look for trusted organic brands.

THE MAGIC OF BLUE-GREEN ALGAE

- PROTEIN POWER

- BOOSTS IMMUNE FUNCTION

- ENERGY BOOSTING

- CLEANSING CHLOROPHYLL

- STRESS RELIEF AND NATURAL ANTIDEPRESSANT

- METAL DETOXING

- BLOOD BUILDING

- LONGEVITY

- WEIGHT LOSS

- GLA SUPER OIL

SPIRULINA HAS A SPIRAL SHAPE, WHICH GIVES IT ITS NAME.

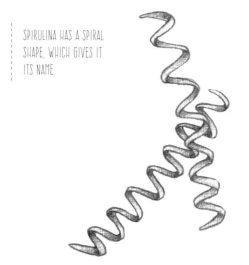

Protein power

The three algae variations covered in this chapter all contain exceptional levels of complete protein. They are the highest protein foods in the world, at 60–75% protein by weight—three times more than meat! The glycoprotein and amino acid peptide forms of protein in algae are easily assimilated, requiring less energy to absorb and utilize compared to animal protein. Repairing tissues and building neurotransmitters can be more easily and swiftly done due to its digestibility. Spirulina yields 200 times more protein per acre than beef and is four times more absorbable than beef, making it better for our bodies and the planet!

Boosts immune function

The blue color in blue-green algae is known as phycocyanin. It boosts immune function by stimulating the production of more stem cells from bone marrow.

Energy boosting

Algae contain both water- and fat-soluble vitamins and are a rich source of vitamin B. All the B vitamins are present, naturally boosting energy levels.

Cleansing chlorophyll

Chlorophyll is the green pigment in algae. It aids in cleansing and detoxifying the body and stimulates blood production, which in turn strengthens the immune system. Chlorella contains more chlorophyll than any other plant.

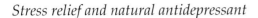

Stress relief and natural antidepressant

Protein-rich superfoods play an important role in reducing stress levels. From these super protein sources our bodies create the neurotransmitters that we need to turn off the stress and turn on the happiness. AFA algae contain the powerful brain-boosting chemical phenylethylamine (PEA). PEA is known as the "love chemical" and naturally allows dopamine levels to rise in the brain, increasing mental concentration and a positive attitude. Studies have shown that PEA plays a significant role in improving conditions such as attention deficit disorder (ADD) and depression. The rich array of amino acids in algae, especially tryptophan, creates a serotonin stress-defense shield in the brain, helping to relieve stress and conquer depression.

Metal detoxing

Numerous studies and research projects have shown that chlorella has a powerful ability to assist the body in breaking down heavy metals and toxins, such as mercury, lead, cadmium, arsenic, pesticides, and herbicides. It has also been shown to help the body remove alcohol from the liver.

Blood building

Algae contain various trace minerals and provide on average four times more calcium than whole milk and fifty times more iron than spinach, effectively correcting anemia and allowing the body to produce energy. Chlorella growth factor (CGF) has been shown to powerfully rebuild nerve and tissue damage.

Longevity

Spirulina in particular contains a powerful combination of antioxidants. Its ORAC (oxygen radical absorbance capacity) value of 61,900 makes it one of the highest of any food! Algae also contain large amounts of betacarotene. Research indicates that the more betacarotene you have in your diet, the longer you will live. Chlorella has more RNA than any other food. RNA is essential in maintaining the longevity of cells.

CHLORELLA CONTAINS GROWTH FACTOR (CGF) ALLOWING IT TO QUADRUPLE EVERY TWENTY-FOUR HOURS. THIS MAKES IT THE FASTEST GROWING FOOD CROP KNOWN.

Weight loss

Algae, with their wide mineral spectrum, are a natural appetite suppressant. They help one to overcome sugar cravings by balancing blood sugar levels and nourishing the body with minerals.

GLA (gamma linolenic acid) super oil

After human breast milk, spirulina is the highest whole food source of the rare oil GLA. GLA has been shown to reduce inflammation, reduce allergies, and foster hormonal and mental development. Ten grams of spirulina provides approximately 131 mg of GLA.

A source of B12?

Blue-green algae do contain the elusive vitamin B12. There is much uncertainty around whether the B12 in algae is usable, since most of the B12 in an analogue form is not absorbable by the human body. While the research is inconclusive, many people are assuming that B12 in the analogue form blocks true B12 absorption, which may not be the case.

What we have managed to piece together is that there are processes in healthy people that actually distinguish between active B12 and the inactive analogues. B12 analogues that are not 100% usable for humans do not really seem to pose a problem. Some research[1] suggests that there is more than enough active B12 in algae: "Figures demonstrate that about 36% of the total corrinoid vitamin B12 activity in spirulina is human active."

It has also been shown that up to 90% of the B12 in regular supplements are analogues too! Experiments show that spirulina has 1,700 times more B12 than eggs, which are considered a reliable source of B12 in spite of its low absorption rate. Just like spirulina, eggs have also been described as potentially blocking the absorption of true B12.

SPIRULINA FED ONE OF THE BIGGEST CITIES IN THE ANCIENT WORLD, MEXICO CITY.

[1] www.veganforum.com/forums/showthread.php?317-B12-and-B12-analogues-in-multivitamins-animal-foods-and-spirulina
www.textfiles.com/food/b12.txt
www.ncbi.nlm.nih.gov/pmc/articles/PMC370297/
www.rawgosia.com/articles/sevenpoints.html

HOW WE USE BLUE-GREEN ALGAE

Spirulina has a unique, strong, salty taste, which some find unpleasant. This is why taking spirulina in tablet form is an easy way to get the benefits without the taste. We regularly take 10–15 spirulina tablets in the morning with a large glass of water.

Spirulina powder can be mixed into fresh juices or smoothies. Start with half a teaspoon and gradually build up to 1–2 teaspoons of spirulina powder daily. A recommended minimum dose is 3 g. It should be taken daily for overall health maintenance. The recipes in this chapter are designed to help mask the algae's intense flavor.

Chlorella is most often sold in tablet form, but can also be added to superfoods drinks as a powder. Three grams is recommended as a maintenance dose. For metal detoxing, 7 g a day is suggested. CGF is an extract of chlorella that can also be used.

There are a few brands of AFA algae available. E3Live has an excellent product that is sold as dried flakes and is easy to add to superfood drinks. Start with 1 g daily and slowly build up to 3 g daily. Therapeutic doses can be as high as 10 g daily. E3Live also has a PEA-concentrated product called BrainON specifically designed for brain health. The Pure Synergy brand offers a magical dried Klamath crystals product that sparkles like emeralds.

See which algae work for your body. Some people prefer one type over another, but they all offer amazing nutrition.

WARNINGS

Algae can be very detoxifying, so it is recommended to start slowly and build up your daily dose over time.

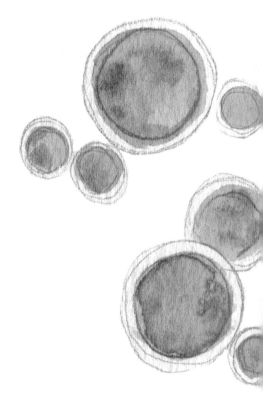

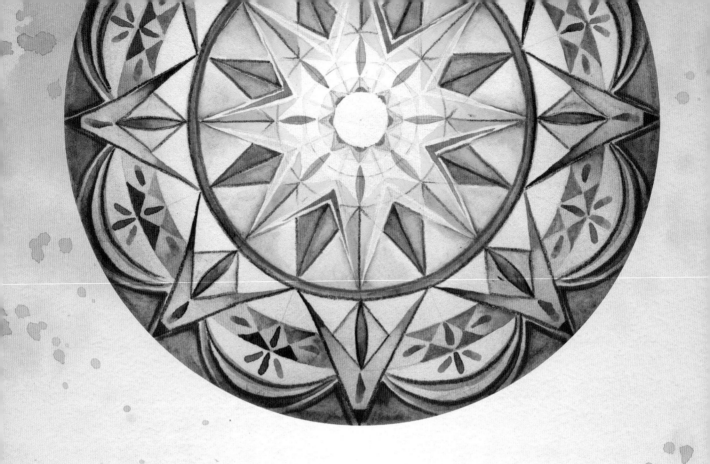

BLUE-GREEN ALGAE RECIPES

—∞—∞—∞———∞——∞—∞—∞—∞———∞—

ALGAE JUICE ∗ SUPER-POWER ALGAE ELIXIR

SUPER-ALKALIZING GREEN JUICE ∗ SUPER-IMMUNE BLUE JUICE

CREAMY MINT SPIRULINA SMOOTHIE ∗ SPIRULINA PEPPERMINT CRISP DESSERT

SPIRULINA LEMON PIE WITH CHOCOLATE CRUST

SUPERFOOD PROTEIN KALE CHIPS ∗ 3-ALGAE HEMP AND CORIANDER PESTO

—∞—∞—∞———∞———∞—∞—∞—∞———∞—

ALGAE JUICE

Take 8–10 oz of fresh fruit juice such as orange juice, grapefruit juice, or apple juice, and add 1 t spirulina powder, chlorella powder, or AFA crystals, with a squeeze of lemon.

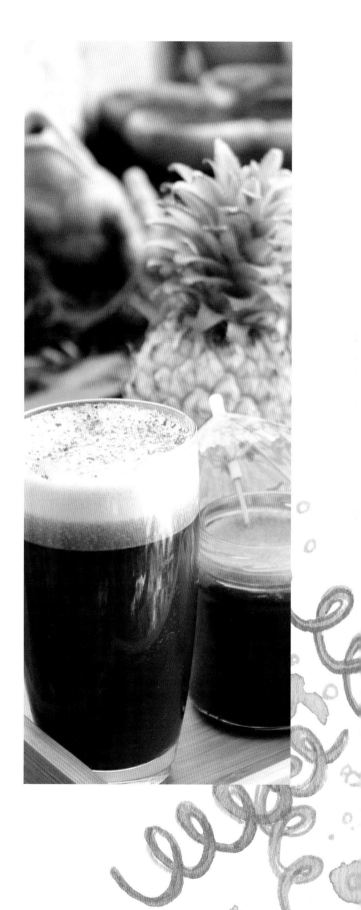

SUPER-POWER ALGAE ELIXIR

Makes 2 C

> 2 C water
> juice of 1 lemon
> 1 T camu camu powder
> 2 T honey
> 1 t spirulina powder or AFA Klamath crystals (or both)
> ½ t E3Live BrainON AFA algae (if available)
> ⅛ t cayenne pepper

For a quick, super-potent algae elixir, blend all the ingredients together and supercharge your system. BrainON is an extract of AFA algae and is high in PEA, which increases concentration and improves mood.

SUPER-ALKALIZING GREEN JUICE

Makes 1 C, dilute with 1 C water to make 2 C

> 1 apple
> 1–2 carrots
> ½ cucumber
> 2 celery stalks
> ½ pineapple
> 5 big leaves spinach or Swiss chard
> 3 big leaves kale
> 1 lemon
> ½–1 t spirulina powder
> 1 t AFA Klamath crystals

Juice all the ingredients and dilute with 1 C water.

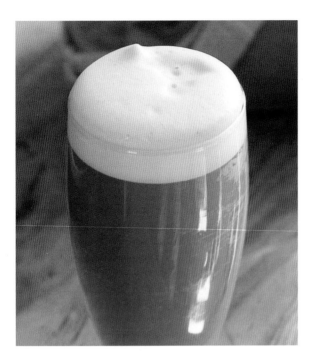

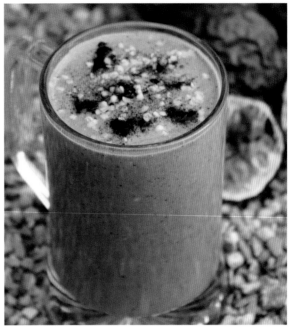

SUPER-IMMUNE BLUE JUICE

Stir a teaspoon of spirulina into a glass of water and allow it to stand overnight—the green pigments will sink to the bottom and the blue pigments will stay suspended, making the water a beautiful bright azure blue color. Slowly pour off the blue water and use in this recipe. Keep the green water for another drink. Alternatively, if you have access to it, phyco-cyanin powder is an extract of the blue pigments.

Makes 3 C

>   2 C blue water
>   1 C coconut kefir, coconut water, or water
>   1 T camu camu powder
>   2 T honey
>   1 handful fresh mint

Blend and enjoy!

CREAMY MINT SPIRULINA SMOOTHIE

Hiding the taste of spirulina in a drink is always a challenge. We were pleasantly surprised with this one: the hemp seeds, the buchu, and the mint make it creamy and minty!

Makes 3 C

>   1 C water
>   2 frozen bananas
>   ½ pineapple or 2 mangoes
>   2 passion fruits
>   ¼ C hemp seeds
>   ⅛ C chia seeds
>   1 T spirulina or algae of your choice
>   1 t buchu powder
>   1 handful fresh mint
>   2 t hemp oil (optional)

Blend everything together and drink.

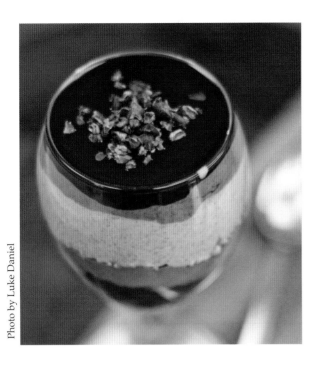

Photo by Luke Daniel

SPIRULINA PEPPERMINT CRISP DESSERT

We've always liked peppermint crisp dessert, which is a peppermint-flavored, crystallized sugar, chocolate treat from my youth. This one is a great alternative in terms of taste and incredible on a nutritional level.

Fills 2 wine glasses, serves 2

> *2 portions of chia omega cream (see page 64)*
> *½ t spirulina*
> *2 drops peppermint essential oil*
> *vanilla buckwheaties (see page 189)*
> *chocolate sauce (see page 229)*
> *a sprinkling of cacao nibs (for decoration)*

Take one portion of chia omega cream and flavor it with the spirulina and peppermint essential oil. Then, in a glass, layer one layer of the plain cream, one layer of the green (peppermint) cream, one layer of the vanilla buckwheaties, then one layer of the chocolate sauce. Repeat until the glass is filled, and top with cacao nibs. The crunch of the vanilla buckwheaties, the green minty cream, and the chocolate sauce combined give that peppermint crisp feel and flavor.

SPIRULINA LEMON PIE WITH CHOCOLATE CRUST

Serves 10–12

For the crust:

> *2 C almonds, soaked*
> *1 C pecans*
> *¼ C raw cacao powder*
> *¼ C mesquite powder*
> *1 t vanilla powder, extract or pod*
> *2 T honey*
> *1 T coconut oil*

For the lemon filling:

> *4 ripe avocados*
> *1 C lemon juice*
> *2 T lemon zest*
> *1 C honey (or ½ C honey and ½ C maple syrup)*
> *½ C coconut oil*
> *1 T spirulina powder*
> *1 t vanilla extract*
> *¼ t Himalayan rock salt*

In a food processor, grind the nuts into a fine, crumbly mixture. Add the remaining crust ingredients and pulse until combined.

Use a quiche tin with removable base or a springform cake tin. Press the mixture into the bottom. Puncture holes into the base using a fork and put it into the fridge while you make the filling.

Blend all the filling ingredients together in a power blender until smooth. Pour into the crust base and refrigerate. Allow to set for one hour.

In this recipe, the avocados provide the bulk for the filling. The key with this tart is to put in enough lemon and honey to offset the flavor of the avocados and spirulina.

Enjoy this green spirulina lemon pie.

SUPERFOOD PROTEIN KALE CHIPS

Fills approximately 5 Excalibur trays (12 x 12in)

5 bunches kale
1 t salt
1 T olive oil

For the algae and hemp garlic green sauce:

1 C warm water
½ C hemp seeds
1 C cashews or macadamia nuts
2–3 garlic cloves
juice of 1 lemon
2 T hemp oil
1 T hemp protein powder
1 t spirulina powder (or AFA Klamath crystals)
1 t kelp powder
1 t salt

This recipe became an instant favorite the first time we tried it!

We find that when we eat kale chips, we can just eat and eat and eat more of them; they are an insatiable snack. However, with the nutrient density of the algae, hemp, and kelp, these kale chips are so deeply nourishing that the body turns off its hunger signals after a short while. Remember—hunger is the body's search for nutrients, and this one is mega-packed with nutrients!

Destalk the kale and place the leaves in a bowl. Sprinkle with the salt and olive oil. Massage through and set aside.

Blend the sauce ingredients together in a blender and pour over the kale. Massage the sauce through the kale, coating it thoroughly. Dehydrate for 12–16 hours.

3-ALGAE HEMP AND CORIANDER PESTO

3 C fresh coriander
2 cloves garlic
⅓ C almonds, soaked
⅓ C sunflower seeds
⅓ C pumpkin seeds
⅓ C hemp seeds
⅔ C olive oil
¼ C hemp oil
juice of 1 lemon
1 T AFA Klamath crystals
½ t spirulina powder
½ t chlorella powder or CGF
½ t kelp powder
½ t Himalayan rock salt

A variation of our original coriander pesto recipe, this one is the real McCoy—loaded with algae, hemp, and kelp.

Place all the ingredients in a food processor or power blender and blend until everything is well combined. Enjoy with a salad, on crackers, or with our kelp noodle pesto dish (see page 164).

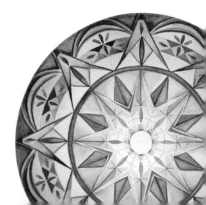

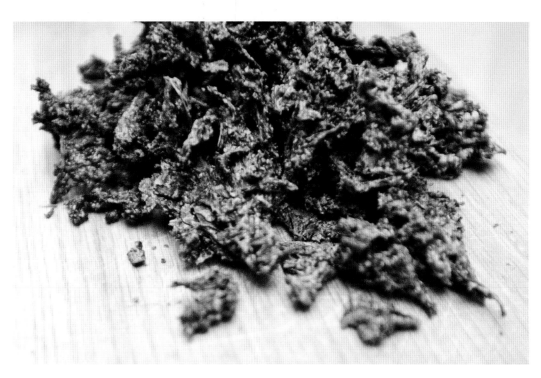

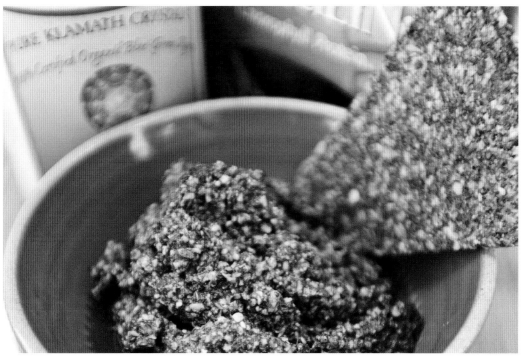

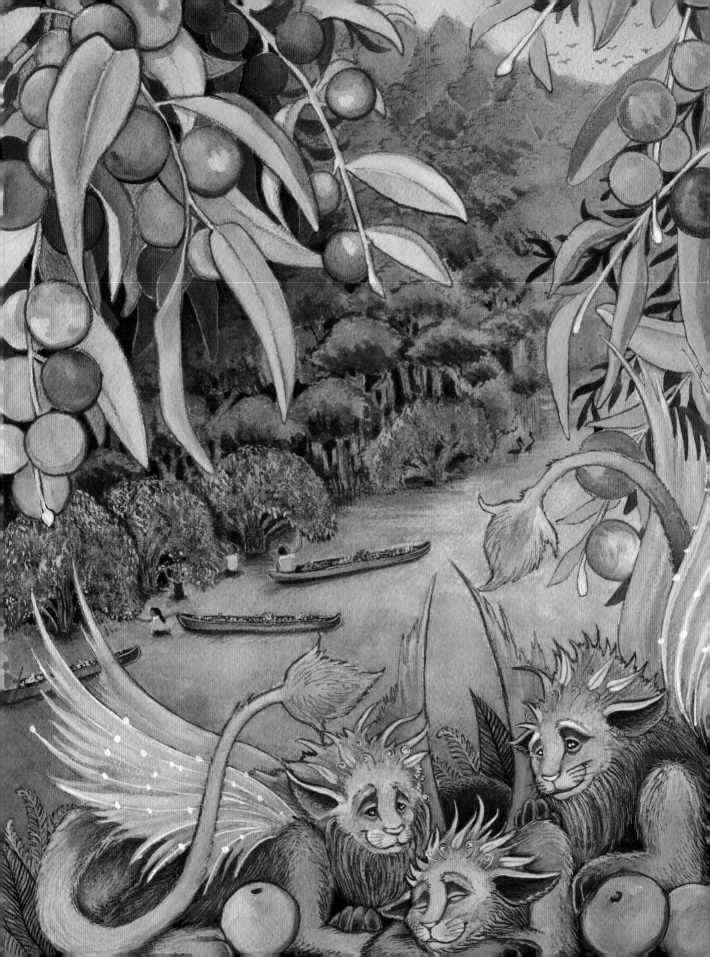

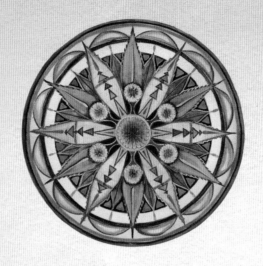

CAMU CAMU

AMAZONIAN VITAMIN C SUPERFRUIT

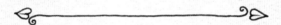

ANTIDEPRESSANT • IMMUNE SYSTEM SUPPORT

NERVOUS SYSTEM PROTECTOR • ANTI-ARTHRITIC

ANTIVIRAL • CALMING • LONGEVITY

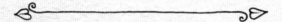

On the banks of the powerful Amazon River,
With roots in the water and leaves all aquiver,
Stand trees sporting berries, which drip from their limbs,
While harvesters pick them, and fill canoes to their brims.
Do they see the sprightly creatures that quickly whizz
Between the branches imparting a tangy fizz
To each berry as they sunkiss it, coax it to ripen,
To strengthen your immunity, your mood to lighten,
To build your body and sharpen your eyes,
To clear your mind and help you grow wise.
Camu camu berry, small, wild, and tart,
We give thanks for the lightness and strength you impart!

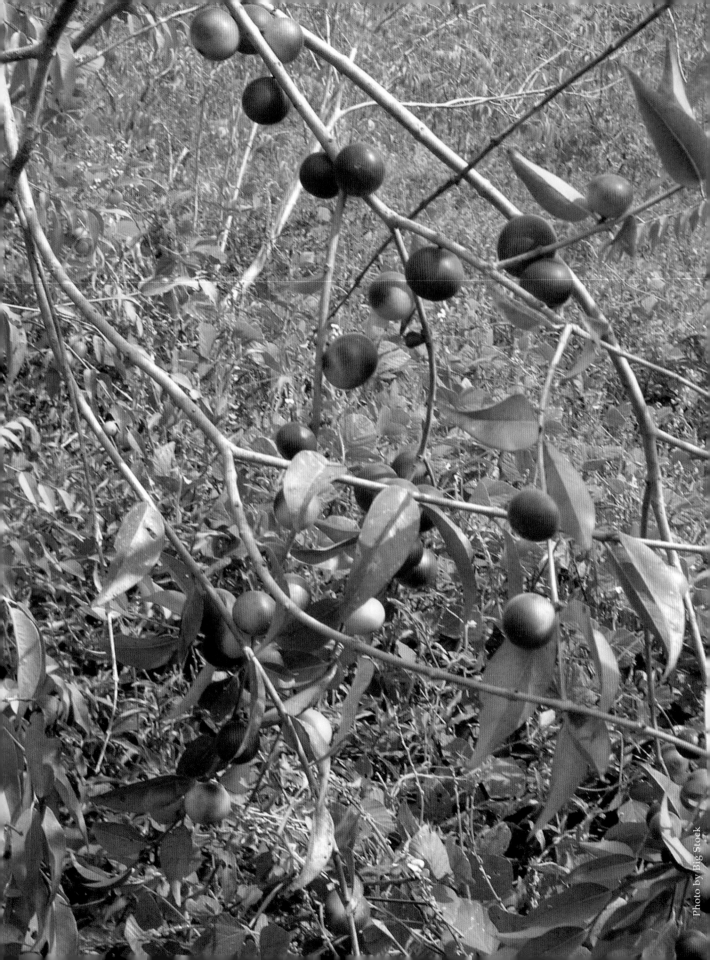

Photo by Big Stock

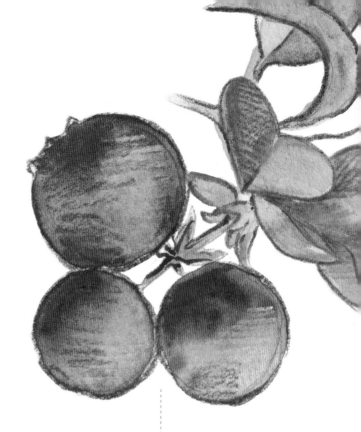

ANCIENT, REVERED SUPERFOOD

Camu camu is a South American bush that grows on the river banks of the Amazon rainforest. It occurs naturally in areas of periodic flooding, such as lowlands around river courses and lakes. The berries of the camu camu bush have been used by Amazonian Indians for thousands of years.

This highly nutritious, small, red fruit is a rich source of phytochemicals and antioxidants that support and enhance health. Camu camu berries are one of the highest sources of vitamin C in the world, containing fifty times more than oranges! Natural plant-source vitamin C is a powerful antioxidant that prevents damage to your DNA caused by free radicals. The berries are also a significant source of potassium, iron, calcium, and vitamin A.

Traditional uses, besides food, include relieving pain, treating infection, and promoting long life.

CAMU CAMU WAS USED BY INDIGENOUS AMAZONIAN CULTURES FOR CENTURIES AS AN IMMUNE TONIC.

CAMU CAMU RECIPES

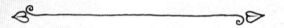

CLEANSING WATERMELON AND CAMU ELIXIR

CAMUNADE * CAMU HONEY

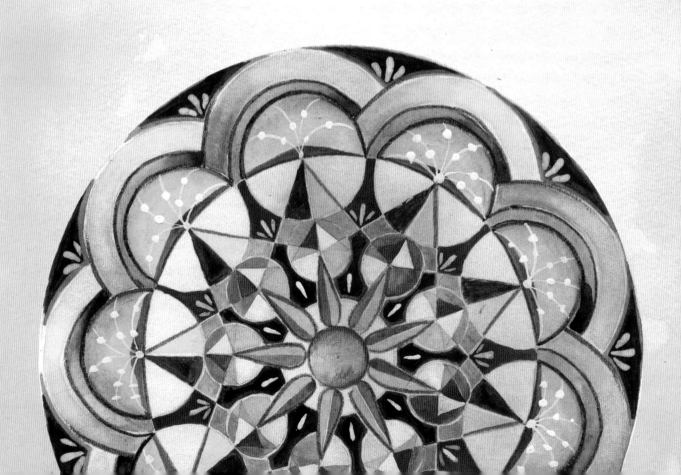

CLEANSING WATERMELON AND CAMU ELIXIR

Makes 1–2 qt

> 1 watermelon
> 2 T camu camu powder
> 1 T honey
> a handful of fresh mint or a cube of fresh ginger
>   (optional)

Blend all the ingredients together. This watermelon and camu combination is a very nourishing, hydrating, and cleansing elixir.

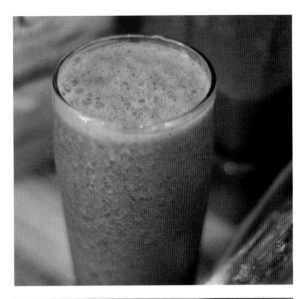

CAMUNADE

This is the way that we use camu camu powder most often.

Makes 2 C

> 2 C water
> 1 T camu camu powder
> 1 T honey
> juice of ½ lemon
> 1 t baobab (optional)
> 10 drops of Concentrace Mineral Solution (a trace
>   mineral supplement) (optional)

Blend ingredients together on low speed in a blender.

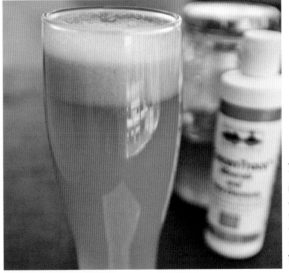

CAMU HONEY
Immune-boosting flu buster

> ½ C honey
> 1 T camu camu powder

Take a small jar of honey, add a tablespoon of camu camu powder, and stir. Eat it straight off the teaspoon as a vitamin C immune-boosting flu buster and sore throat soother.

You'll also find camu camu in these recipes:

Aloe citrus (see page 27)
Aloe and grapefruit skin cleanser (see page 29)
Bao sorbet (see page 39)
The original sherbet (see page 39)
Goji winter citrus (see page 49)
Super-power algae elixir (see page 97)
Super-immune blue juice (see page 98)

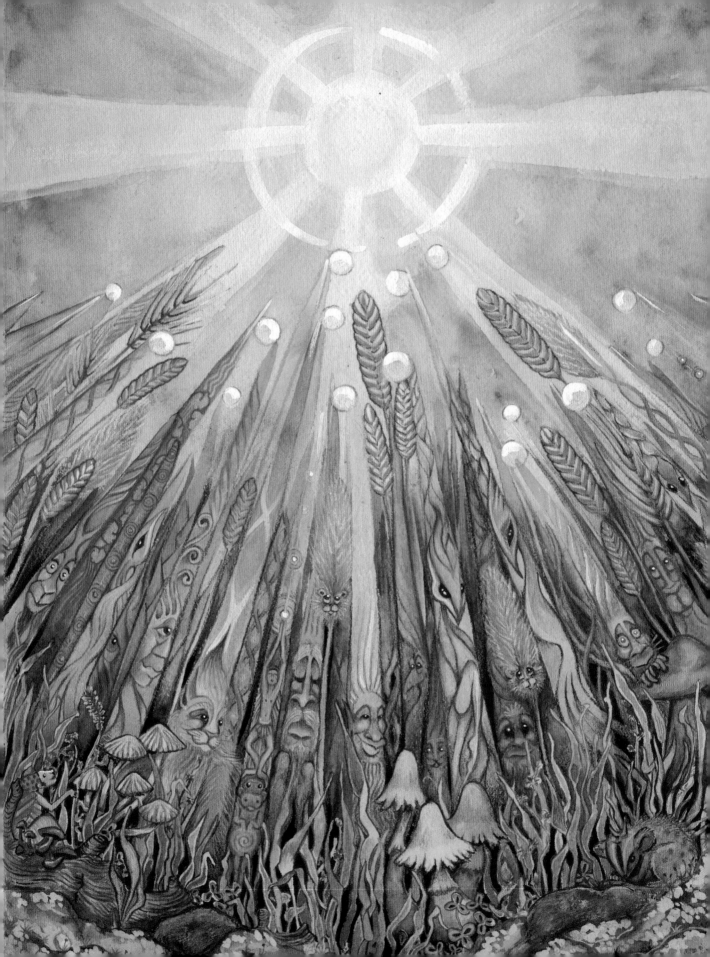

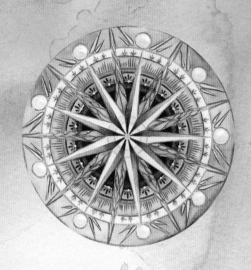

GRASSES AND MICROGREENS
ALKALIZING NUTRIENT POWERHOUSE

·»⊪———————————————⊪«·

NUTRIENT POWERHOUSES · DIGESTIVE HEALTH · CLEANSING
PROTEIN BUILDING · LONGEVITY ANTIOXIDANTS
BLOOD OXYGENATING · ANTICARCINOGENIC · ALKALIZING

·»⊪———————————————⊪«·

Under the ground lies a network of roots
A labyrinth out of which sprout shining green shoots
A smooth sheer blade that streams towards the sun
To gather the light from which grasses are spun.
Sun photosynthesis: green chlorophyll.
Soil from which every mineral is pulled.
The largest beasts of the land eat grass
It builds their bodies, and makes up their mass
Enormous elephant! Regal horse!
Rhino and Eland; all eat grass, of course.
The tiniest creatures rely on grass too.
Imagine being tiny. Imagine it's you
In a maze of green walkways, sun filtering down,
A mosaic of light, and on each grass blade's crown
Hangs a perfect orb of dew like a glass chandelier
A sparkling world, with a mind bright and clear.

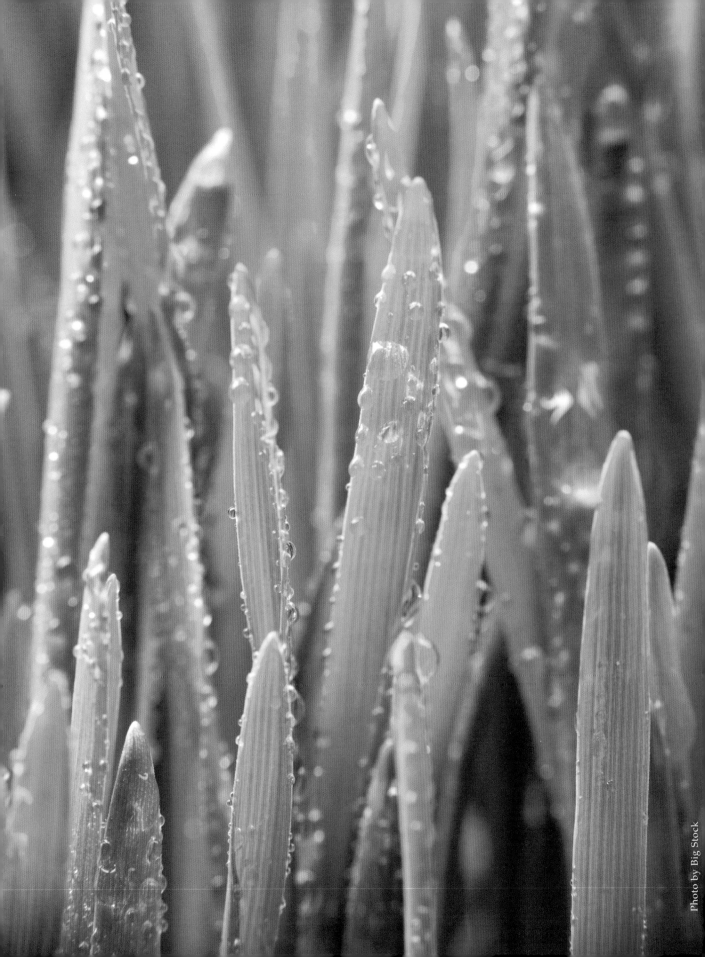

ANCIENT, REVERED SUPERFOOD

When it comes to alkalization, grasses are key. Chlorophyll-rich grasses are like shots of bottled sunshine, inhibiting disease-causing bacteria while alkalizing, cleansing, and energizing the cells. Grasses are some of the few plants that can absorb and pull up all the minerals present in the soil in which they are grown, making them particularly nutrient dense. Drinking wheatgrass or barleygrass juice is one of the best and quickest ways to alkalize the body. Wheatgrass and barleygrass are either dried and powdered to make supplements, or picked fresh and juiced. As young grasses, wheat and barley are closer to vegetables than grains in composition. While eating too much wheat and wheat products is not advisable—and allergenic for some—wheatgrass juice is an excellent addition to your diet.

In the 1960s, American health educator and raw-food advocate Ann Wigmore used wheatgrass to help cure her own intractable colitis. She went on to form the famous Hippocrates Health Institute in Florida, treating various conditions using large amounts of fresh wheatgrass juice, which they still do to this day.

There is very little nutritional difference between wheatgrass and barleygrass. You can drink freshly cut wheatgrass or barleygrass juice, usually sold as "shots" at health food stores, or get grasses in powder or tablet form. Dried grasses are certainly easier to handle than fresh. However, fresh grass juice contains healthful enzymes not found in dried grass powder and, overall, has a higher nutrient profile.

Growing your own wheatgrass or barleygrass is easy and fun. You will need a masticating juicer to be able to extract the potent juice. Young grasses are also referred to as "microgreens." Sunflower greens are another microgreen that are extremely nutritious to juice as well as delicious to eat. It takes only seven to ten days to grow your own!

GRASSES ARE THE ONLY PLANTS THAT CONTAIN ALL THE MINERALS IN THE SOIL.

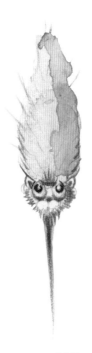

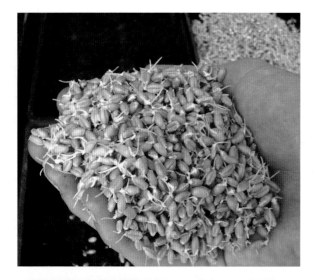

SOIL-GROWN MICROGREENS

Microgreens such as wheatgrass, barleygrass, and sunflower greens are grown in soil trays.

How to grow soil-based sprouts:

- Buy trays and organic growing soil from a nursery.
- Fill the trays with soil.
- Soak wheat, barley, or sunflower seeds overnight.
- Drain them in the morning and allow them to stand in a bowl for twenty-four to forty-eight hours. Small tails will sprout.
- Place the seeds on top of the soil, cover with another thin layer of soil, and lightly water them.
- Place them in an area that gets either morning or afternoon sun (midday summer sun will burn the young shoots) and water daily.
- Harvest the wheatgrass or barleygrass after seven to ten days and juice them.
- Harvest the sunflower sprouts after seven to ten days and either juice them or eat them in salads.

To make sure you are growing the most potent microgreens that you can, water the soil with a solution of sea salt rich in trace minerals. Take Himalayan rock salt and make a saltwater solution of one part salt to two hundred parts water. Water the sprouts from day four to day seven with this saltwater solution. Alternatively, get seawater (from a clean source, preferably a few miles out to sea) and make the solution from one part seawater to twenty parts freshwater and proceed as before. You will have the healthiest-looking, best-tasting, most nutritious microgreens around.

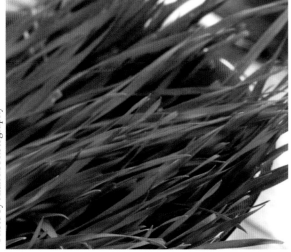

Photo by Alan M Photography

THE MAGIC OF GRASSES AND MICROGREENS

NUTRIENT POWERHOUSES

DIGESTIVE HEALTH

CLEANSING

PROTEIN BUILDING

LONGEVITY ANTIOXIDANTS

BLOOD OXYGENATING

ANTICARCINOGENIC

ALKALIZING

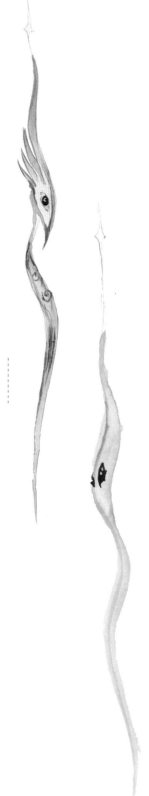

EVEN THOUGH THE WORD "WHEAT" IS IN ITS NAME, WHEATGRASS IS GLUTEN-FREE

Nutrient powerhouses

Grasses are the mineral miners of the plant kingdom, containing over ninety minerals. They are some of the only plants that can absorb all the minerals present in the soil where they grow. It is said that just 1 oz of freshly squeezed wheatgrass juice (a wheatgrass shot) is equivalent in nutritional value to 2.2 lb of green leafy vegetables.

Digestive health

Grasses contain essential enzymes to support digestion. They stimulate the release of digestive HCl (hydrochloric acid), allowing greater absorption of food. It is reported that this allows the reduction of graying hair through greater mineral uptake in the digestive system.

Cleansing

Grasses are also highly regarded for their ability to cleanse the blood, organs, and gastrointestinal tract. High in saponins, grasses offer excellent support to the lymphatic system, helping to carry away thousands of toxins from the cells of the body. This extreme cleansing effect is what can make people feel nauseated when first trying fresh grass juice.

Protein building

The largest land animals eat grass. Think of cows, elephants, and rhinoceroses. Where did they get all the protein to build such huge bodies? Grass. Grass is a complete protein containing nineteen amino acids, the building blocks of protein. The astonishingly high amino acid content in grass is why many bodybuilders and gym-goers are now incorporating it into their daily routine.

Longevity antioxidants

Grasses contain the super-antioxidant, superoxide dismutase (SOD), which is found in all body cells and is known for its ability to lessen the effect of radiation and slow cellular aging. Nitrogen reductase and a number of C-glycosylflavones with documented antioxidant effects have been isolated from grasses.

Blood oxygenating

Chlorophyll is the plant equivalent of the oxygen-carrying red pigment hemoglobin in red blood cells. Grass juice helps your body to build red blood cells, which carry oxygen to every cell.

Anticarcinogenic

In 1931, Otto Warburg won the Nobel prize for his cancer research, which stated: "Cancer is caused by weakened cell respiration due to a lack of oxygen at a cellular level." More chlorophyll equals more oxygen. Many health clinics worldwide, including the Hippocrates Health Institute in Florida, use grass juice as a primary therapy in treating cancer. Cancer thrives in anaerobic and acidic conditions. Grasses, which oxygenate and alkalize, are therefore effective preventative measures. Recent studies show that grass juice has a powerful ability to fight tumors without the usual toxicity of the drugs that are used to inhibit cell-destroying agents.

Alkalizing

Research has shown that the Western lifestyle is causing an over-acidification in people. Acidity creates inflammation, puffiness, water retention, and stiffness and breeds harmful bacteria, parasites, and mold. Green foods are the most potent sources of alkalizing nutrients. People worldwide are reporting the miraculous healing effect of an alkaline diet.

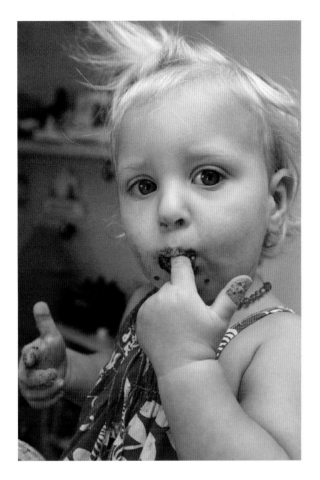
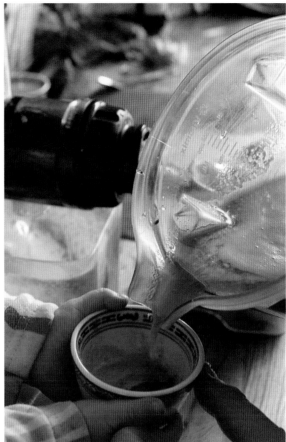

HOW WE USE THE GRASSES

Out of all the superfoods, the grasses are the ones closest to being superherbs, as they cannot be consumed in large quantities because of their detoxing effects. Those who have been on a clean diet for a few years find they can enjoy a much higher dose. We often use up to five heaped tablespoons in a green smoothie.

Fresh wheatgrass or barleygrass is widely available as shots in health stores and juice bars. A shot can be drunk daily, but beware the detox effect. If the fresh juice makes you feel nauseated, rather try the powder for a few weeks before going back to the juice. The powder is less detoxifying and gentler on the system.

There are many brands of grass powders available on the market now at very affordable prices. Look out for a certified organic brand that is free from fillers. Make sure it is the powder of grass juice and not just the whole grass powder, which may contain a lot of indigestible fiber.

Grass powders are easy to add into most superfood drinks and fresh vegetable juices. We often add them to raw chocolates, a great way to get them into unwilling kids! Raw cacao hides the green taste amazingly well. Make a raw cacao superfood smoothie and add in green powders—you may not even notice it!

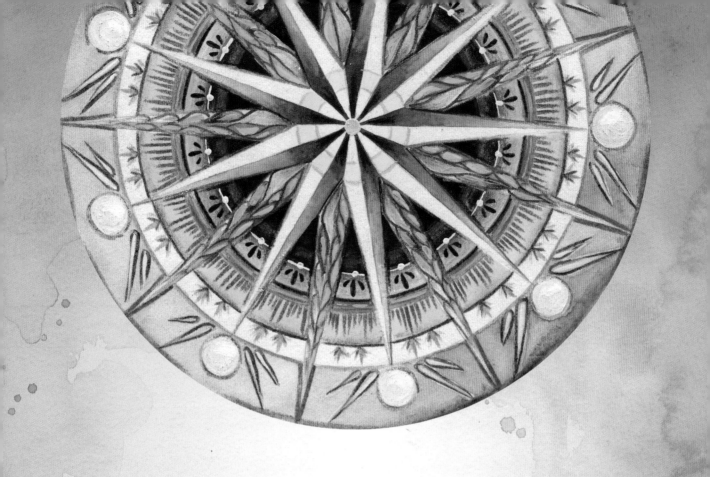

GRASSES AND MICROGREENS RECIPES

·›»‖─────────────────────────‖«·

JUICE POWDERS * WHEATGRASS JUICE SHOTS

THE GRASS IS GREENER * SUNFLOWER SPROUT JUICE

MICROGREEN SALAD

·›»‖─────────────────────────‖«·

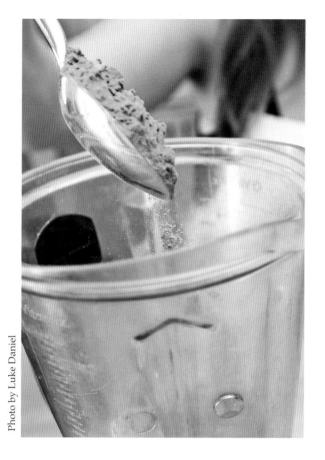

Photo by Luke Daniel

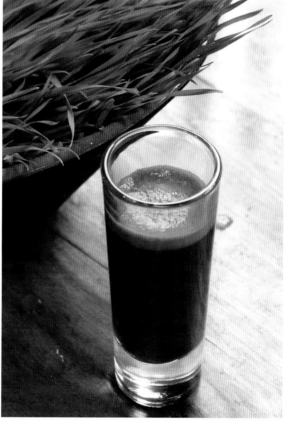

Photo by Alan M Photography

JUICE POWDERS

The absolute simplest way to add grasses to your diet is to get a tub of grass juice powder, such as wheatgrass or barleygrass juice powder or a combination thereof, and place it in a prominent place in your kitchen. Add a tablespoon (or more or less depending on what you find palatable) to your juices to power them up.

WHEATGRASS JUICE SHOTS

Makes 4–5 shots (1 oz each)

1 tray wheatgrass

Cut the grass just above the soil, and juice using a masticating juicer. (A centrifugal juicer will not juice wheatgrass.)

It is best to drink your wheatgrass as soon as it has been juiced, for maximum potency.

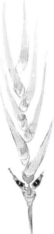

Grasses and Microgreens Recipes   121

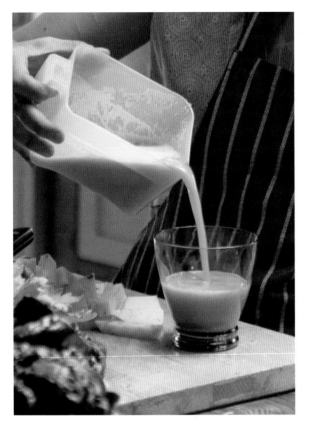
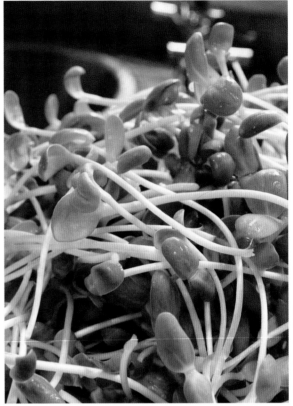

Photos by Alan M Photography

THE GRASS IS GREENER

It is said that one shot of wheatgrass is equivalent to two plates of vegetables.

While many people find neat wheatgrass quite hard to stomach, most find this version much more manageable. The health benefits of juicing wheatgrass are enormous. It's incredibly detoxifying and alkalizing for the body.

Makes 1 C, dilute with the same quantity of water to make 2 C

> *1 apple*
> *½ lemon*
> *1 tray wheatgrass*
> *¾ in ginger*

Juice all the ingredients.

SUNFLOWER SPROUT JUICE

Makes 1 C, dilute with the same quantity of water to make 2 C

> *1 apple*
> *1 carrot*
> *1 lemon*
> *½ tray sunflower sprouts*

Add ½ tray of wheatgrass to this concoction to elevate it to supreme health juice status!

Juice all the ingredients and drink.

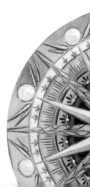

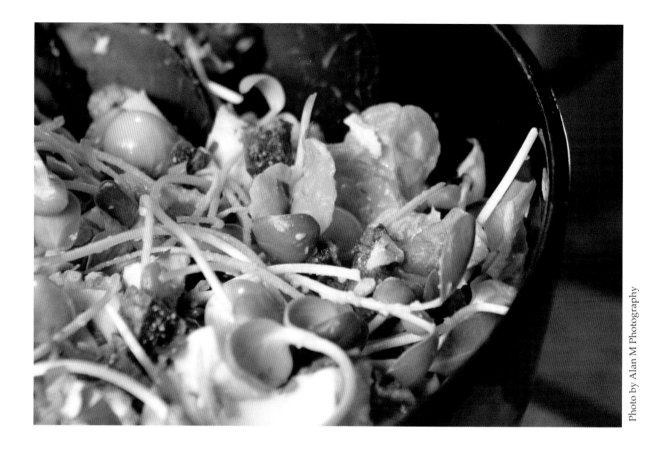

Photo by Alan M Photography

MICROGREEN SALAD

Sunflower sprout salads are still one of the best ways to consume green leafy vegetables as a meal. This is my favorite microgreen salad from our first recipe book, *Rawlicious*.

Grate the carrots and cabbage first. Combine the carrots, cabbage, sunflower greens, sprouts, figs, cherry tomatoes, and walnuts. Top with the avocado and gooseberries. Garnish with the parsley.

Optional: Drizzle with a simple salad dressing of ¼ C olive oil, ⅛ C hemp oil, juice of 1 lemon, and 2 T honey.

Serves 4

2 carrots
½ baby cabbage
1 C sunflower greens
1 C mixed sprouts
a sprinkling of chopped
*   dried figs*
½ C cherry tomatoes
1 handful walnuts
1–2 avocados, diced
1 handful gooseberries
parsley, finely chopped, for
*   garnish*

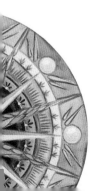

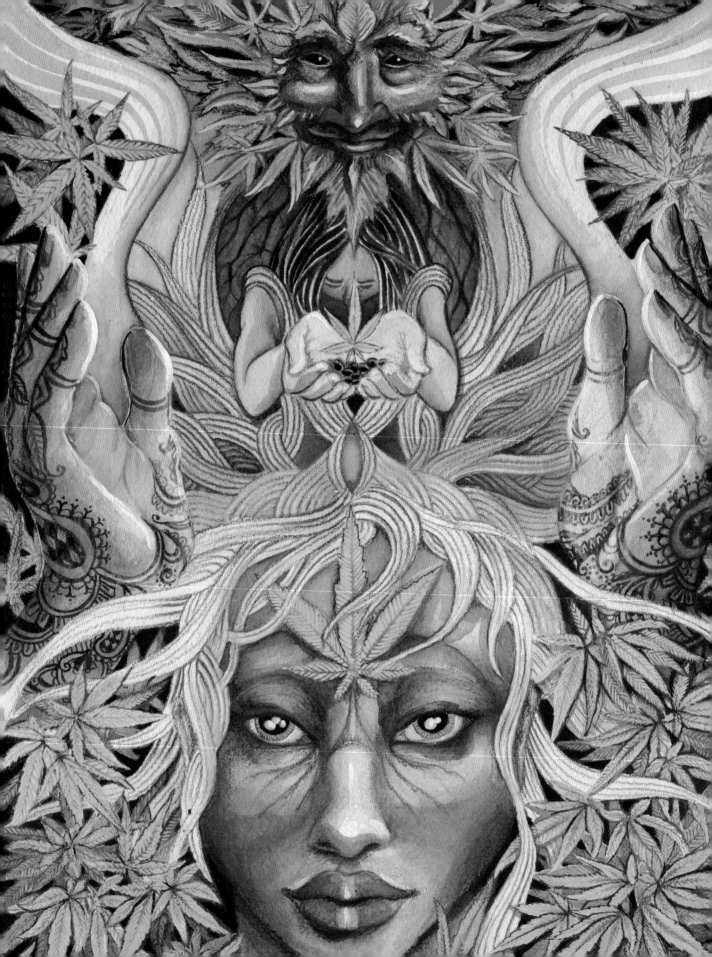

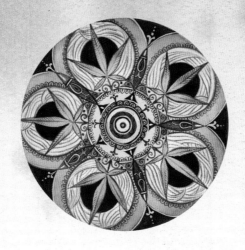

HEMP

ALKALIZING PROTEIN-RICH SUPERFOOD

PROTEIN RICH * IMMUNE SYSTEM SUPPORTIVE

OMEGA-3 RICH * HORMONE BALANCING

LIVER SUPPORTING * DIGESTIVE HEALTH

Have you ever sat still, all surrounded by leaves
And listened acutely while the plant kingdom breathes?
Have you ever closed your eyes, put your hands on the ground
And for a moment felt yourself melt into the surrounds?
Remember, remember, our age-old connection,
The eyes of knowing, the hands of protection,
The vegetal realm, so much generously offered
All that we could need, so willingly proffered.
Hemp: versatile, abundant, sustainable,
Harmonious living made easily attainable.
Long fibrous locks that coil like rope,
Or probe the soil seeking a harvest of hope
A five-fingered leaf like a beckoning hand,
A shepherdess holding the fat of the land.

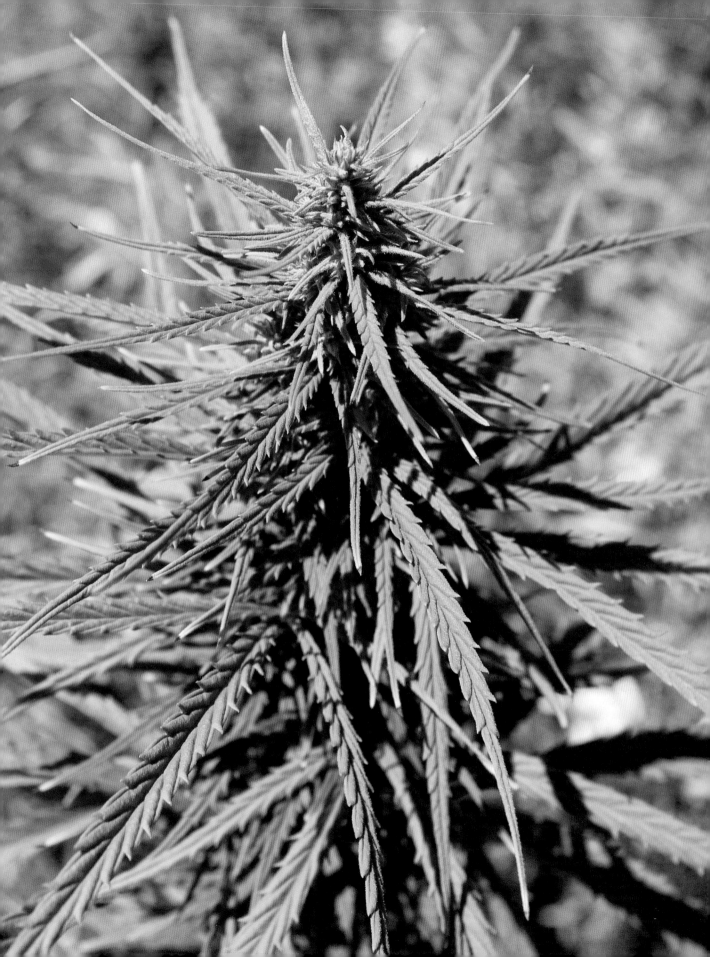

ANCIENT, REVERED SUPERFOOD

Hemp can provide all that is needed to live. It is quite possibly the plant with the closest historical relationship with humans. Its famous five leaves give us an indication of its purpose: to support the five-pointed figure of the human being. Its fiber is used to make clothes, building materials, and fabrics of all kinds. Columbus's sails were made of hemp, the Declaration of Independence was drafted on hemp paper, and, as a highly revered food source, hemp can be traced back thousands of years to cultures the world over. Hemp as a sustainable resource is finally making a reappearance!

Hemp seeds contain all the essential amino acids and fatty acids and are considered to be a complete food. Not only are the leaves delicious to juice, but they are also a powerful antifungal. Hemp seeds seem almost engineered for human compatibility, providing us with the perfect ratio of essential omega oils. Seeds and leaves alike are alkaline and highly nutritious.

As a medicine, the active components—cannabinoids—have been shown to dissolve cancer cells (curing cancer), allow pain relief, prevent Alzheimer's disease, and balance blood sugar levels. As a spiritual sacrament, it has been used by traditions and cultures around the world to reconnect people to the subtle.

Only in the last eighty years has hemp been demonized by propaganda. However, times have changed, and we are once more opening up to our profound link to this plant.

THE WORD "CANVAS" COMES FROM THE MIDDLE ENGLISH WORD "CANEVAS," WHICH COMES FROM THE LATIN WORD "CANNABIS."

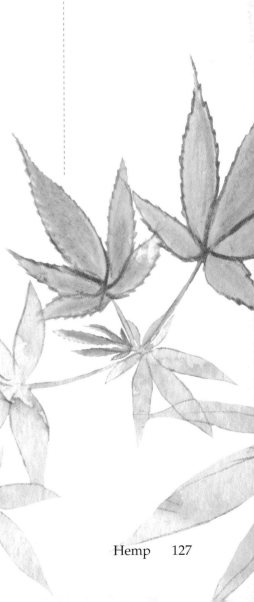

Hemp conspiracy

In the 1930s, corporate gas, cotton, and wood paper interests in the United States created one of the greatest media conspiracies of the century. They manipulated a fear frenzy linking hemp to marijuana. Subsequent drug acts made no distinction between the plants and all but destroyed the US hemp industry. Many countries worldwide have now realized the folly in this and have legalized the growing of hemp for food and fiber, including the United Kingdom, Germany, Canada, and China.

Hemp everything

Hemp is such an easy plant to grow. It requires no herbicides and is able to survive in almost any climate, producing up to three times as much fiber per acre as cotton. Besides food and fiber for textiles, hemp has an astonishing number of uses. In 1941, Henry Ford produced a car made with a hemp resin body that ran on hemp-ethanol fuel! Other uses of hemp include cosmetics, paper, plastics, and building materials. Our friend Tony built his entire house from hemp, including all the furnishings!

Hemp food

Hemp seeds are the part of the plant mainly used for food, although hemp leaves are some of the most nutrient-dense greens known and are great in salads and juices. The seeds can be eaten whole, or ground down into a powder. Hemp food is usually sold as hemp protein powder, shelled seeds, or hemp oil. The protein powder is rich in fiber and protein, the shelled seeds are rich in protein and good oils, and the oil is cold-pressed from the seeds and rich in omega-3s.

At 30% protein content, hemp protein powder is the answer for anyone looking for a raw, vegan, and organic muscle builder and energy booster. The seeds are essential for overall health maintenance, as they contain a wide array of nutrients, antioxidants, and fiber. Hemp oil is a great-tasting food oil used like olive oil. It may contain anticarcinogenic cannabinoids such as CBD but is free of the psychoactive THC.

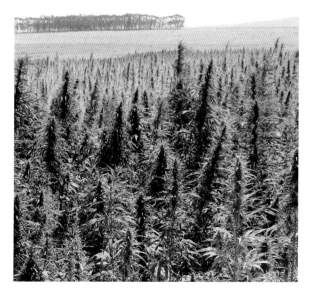

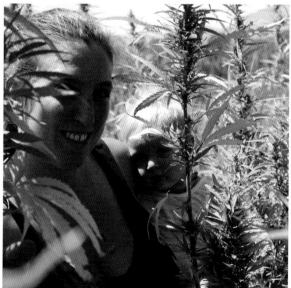

HOW WE USE HEMP

Shelled hemp seeds can be eaten as they are, straight out of the box—they have a mild nutty flavor. They can be added to smoothies or blended into a delicious hemp milk, which can be used as a smoothie base. Sprinkle the seeds onto soups, cereals, or fresh fruit to add more great nutrition to your meal. Our favorite way of using them is to sprinkle them over salads. Take 1–3 T daily or more just following exercise. Hemp seeds are a completely safe and gentle food, and up to 5.25 oz can be eaten a day. It's one of Katara's favorite foods, and you can make an excellent hemp milk for children using this nutrient-rich seed.

Hemp seeds will *not* get you high, as they do not contain THC. Due to their heat-sensitive EFA composition, it is best not to use them in high-temperature cooking.

Hemp oil can be used exactly as is, drizzled onto salads, added into smoothies, or blended into salad dressings.

Hemp protein powder is best used as an addition to smoothies, snack bars, and other savory options (check out our hemp burger recipe in this section).

HEMP PAPER CAN BE RECYCLED UP TO SEVEN TIMES, WOOD PULP PAPER CAN BE RECYCLED FOUR TIMES.

ONE ACRE OF USABLE HEMP FIBER IS EQUAL TO THE USABLE FIBER OF FOUR ACRES OF TREES OR TWO ACRES OF COTTON.

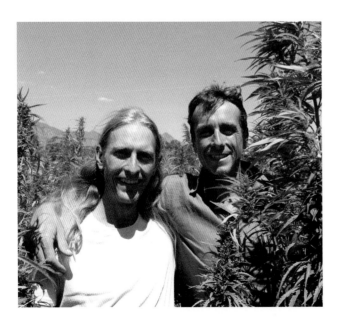

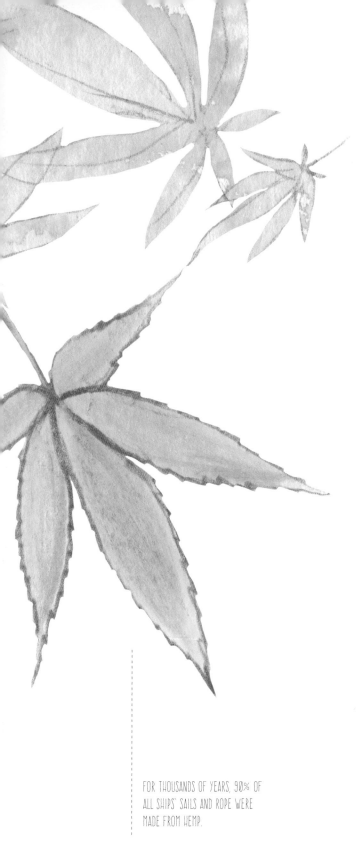

THE MAGIC OF HEMP

- PROTEIN RICH
- IMMUNE SYSTEM SUPPORTIVE
- OMEGA-3 RICH
- HORMONE BALANCING
- LIVER SUPPORTING
- DIGESTIVE HEALTH

Protein rich

Hemp seeds contain all twenty known amino acids, the building blocks of protein, including the nine essential amino acids (EAAs) that our bodies cannot produce. Hemp seeds contain 30% pure digestible protein, providing readily available amino acids for building and repairing tissue. Approximately 65%

FOR THOUSANDS OF YEARS, 90% OF ALL SHIPS' SAILS AND ROPE WERE MADE FROM HEMP.

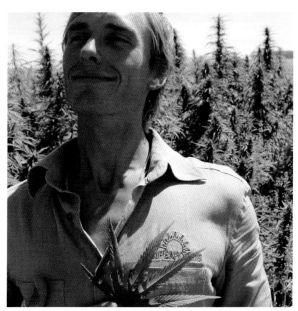

of the protein in hemp seeds is made up of the globulin protein edestin, the most potent protein of any plant source, which is found only in hemp seed. Edestin aids digestion, is relatively phosphorus-free, and is considered to be the backbone of the cell's DNA. The other one third of hemp seed protein is albumin, another high-quality globulin protein similar to that found in egg whites. Hemp protein is free of the trypsin inhibitors that block protein absorption and free of oligosaccharides, which cause stomach upset and gas.

Immune system supportive

The globulin edestin in hemp seed closely resembles the globulin in blood plasma, and is compatible with the human digestive system. It is vital to the maintenance of a healthy immune system and is also used to manufacture antibodies.

Omega-3 rich

The oil from the seeds contains significant amounts of omega-3 and omega-6 EFAs, in a unique, near-perfect ratio for human nutritional needs. The EFAs' powerful antioxidant and anti-inflammatory properties have been shown to help protect the skin from the inside, burn excess body fat, reduce the threat of heart disease, feed the brain and eyes, and support both cell metabolism and the immune system. One tablespoon (0.5 oz) per day of hemp seed oil easily fulfills human daily requirements for EFAs. Skin regeneration and hydration of dry mature skin are enhanced through the use of hemp oil. It increases skin elasticity and water retention capacity in tissues.

REFUSING TO GROW HEMP IN AMERICA DURING THE 17TH AND 18TH CENTURIES WAS AGAINST THE LAW.

Hormone balancing

Hemp oil is the only edible seed that contains GLA. GLA is the precursor for the production of the protective and calming prostaglandin PGE1, which helps regulate hormonal balance and support menopausal health.

Liver supporting

Albumin is a protein manufactured by the liver that is supportive of liver and kidney health. Hemp seed is also a good source of lecithin, which is known to be brain building and liver supportive.

Digestive health

The fiber in hemp seeds is excellent for maintaining overall digestive and colon health.

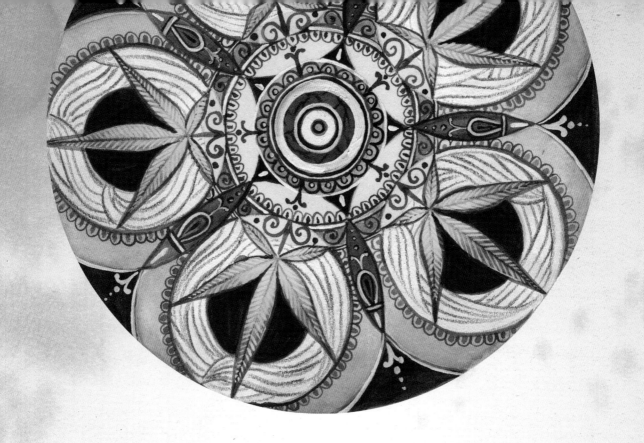

HEMP RECIPES

———◆———

QUEEN OF GREEN HEMP SMOOTHIE * HEMP MILK * HEMP CHEESE
HEMPINI–HEMP BUTTER * HEMP GARLIC WHITE SAUCE
SIMPLE HEMP OIL SALAD DRESSING * HEMP GODDESS GREEN SALAD DRESSING
SALAD SPRINKLE * HEMP BURGERS * HEMP ONION BREAD

———◆———

QUEEN OF GREEN HEMP SMOOTHIE

Green smoothies are an exceptionally good way to get more alkalizing greens into the body. This one has double the power, with the hemp seeds and hemp protein powder adding extra nutritional goodness.

Makes 3 C

> *2 C water*
> *1 apple*
> *1 banana*
> *6 spinach leaves*
> *juice of 1 large lemon*
> *2 T hemp seeds*
> *1 T hemp protein powder*

Blend and drink.

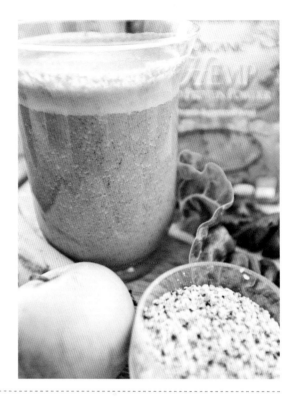

HEMP MILK

Hemp seeds are loaded with good omega oils. We use this simple milk recipe everywhere—over breakfasts, in smoothies, as a basis for ice creams, and so on. Hemp seeds vary from batch to batch, and on occasion they can be a bit bitter. If so, just add a little extra honey to sweeten them up.

Makes 2½ C

> *2 C water*
> *½ C hemp seeds*
> *1 T honey*
> *½ t vanilla powder, extract, or pod*

Blend and enjoy.

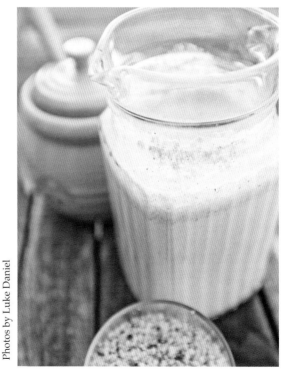

Photos by Luke Daniel

Hemp Recipes   133

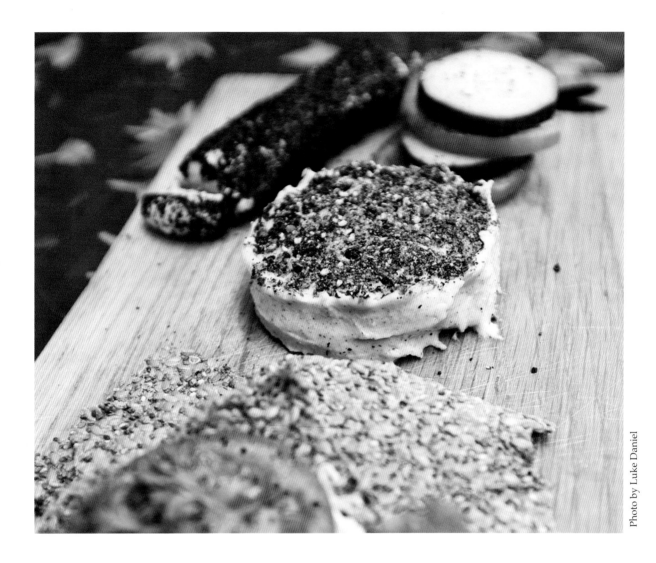

Photo by Luke Daniel

HEMP CHEESE

Makes 2–3 cheese logs or rounds

1 C hemp seeds
1 C macadamia nuts
2 cloves garlic
juice of 1 lemon
1 t salt
¼ t black pepper
dried herbs or ground pepper
  for rolling into nut log or
  round

Soak nuts and hemp seeds together for one hour and then strain, discarding the soak water. Blend in a power blender together with remaining ingredients until smooth. You will need to use a tamper to get the smooth consistency. Wet your hands slightly and roll the cheese into nut log shapes or cheese rounds. Dip or roll in dried herbs or black pepper. Totally delicious served with crackers!

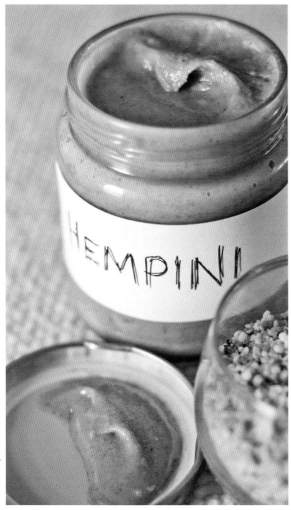

Photos by Luke Daniel

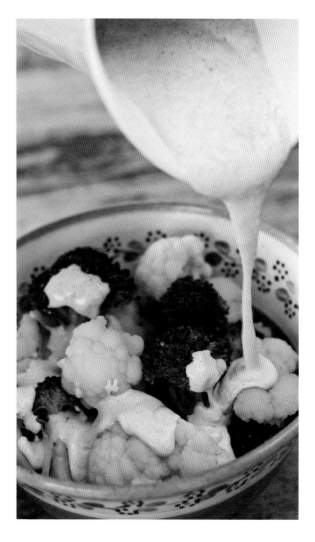

HEMPINI—HEMP BUTTER

Move over, peanut butter; try this superfood hempini instead!

Makes 17 oz

> *2 C hemp seeds*
> *1 C macadamia nuts*
> *¼ C cacao butter*
> *¼ t salt*

Blend in power blender until smooth. Store in a glass jar.

HEMP GARLIC WHITE SAUCE

Makes 1 ½ C

> *1 C warm water*
> *½ C hemp seeds*
> *½ C cashews*
> *2–3 garlic cloves*
> *juice of 1 lemon*
> *2 T hemp oil*
> *1 t salt*

Blend in a power blender. This tastes amazing drizzled over fresh or slightly steamed veggies and can also be used as the sauce for coating kale chips.

Hemp Recipes   135

SIMPLE HEMP OIL SALAD DRESSING

Makes ½ C

> ¼ C hemp oil
> ¼ C olive oil
> 3 T apple cider vinegar
> 2 T honey
> 1 clove garlic, chopped
> 1 t tamari
> ½ t salt

Hemp oil has the perfect ratio between omega-3, -6 and -9 for human consumption, so make sure to use it in your salad dressings.

Combine all the ingredients in a glass jar and shake vigorously.

HEMP GODDESS GREEN SALAD DRESSING

Makes ½ C

> ¼ C hemp oil
> ¼ C olive oil
> juice of 1 lemon
> 2 T honey
> 2 T Rosendal vinegar
> 1 t hemp protein powder
> ½ t spirulina powder
> ½ t salt
> 2 T hemp seeds (optional)

This recipe, with the extra hemp powder and spirulina, has raised the bar on the nutritional profile of a simple salad dressing.

Blend on low speed until well combined.

SALAD SPRINKLE

Fills 8–10 oz jar

> ½ C hemp seeds
> ¼ C sunflower seeds
> ¼ C pumpkin seeds
> ¼ C chia seeds
> 1 T powdered sea vegetable
> 1 T salt
> 1 t kelp powder
> ⅓ C dried pitted olives
>   (optional addition)

If you take this salad sprinkle and an avocado with you to any restaurant, you can spruce up a simple salad inconspicuously in less than a minute!

Put all the ingredients together in a jar and shake thoroughly.

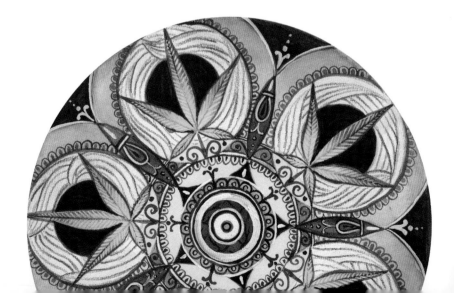

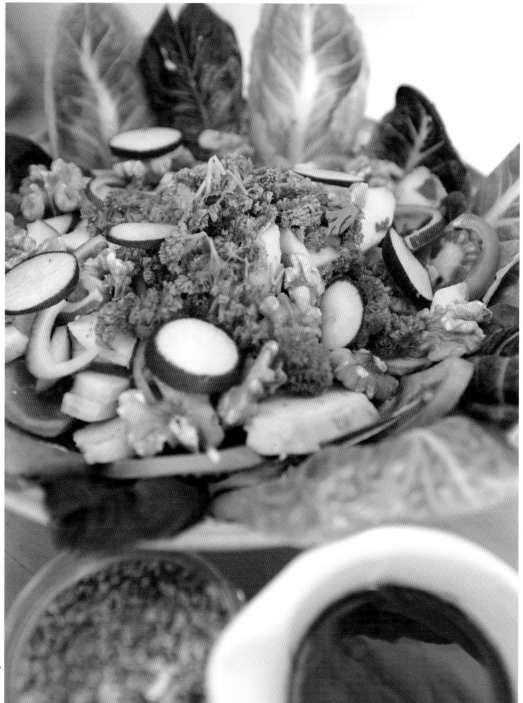

HEMP BURGERS

Makes 16 patties

- *½ C hemp seeds*
- *½ C sunflower seeds*
- *½ C almonds*
- *½ C dried olives*
- *¼ C sundried tomatoes*
- *2 large brown mushrooms*
- *3 carrots*
- *2 medium zucchini squashes*
- *1 onion*
- *½ avocado*
- *¼ C hemp protein powder*
- *3 garlic cloves*
- *2 T chia seeds*
- *2 T tamari*
- *1 T hemp oil*
- *1 T miso*
- *1 t salt*
- *2 C tightly packed, mixed fresh herbs such as parsley, coriander, rosemary, sage (you could use dried herbs, but fresh is much better)*

Soak the seeds, nuts, olives, and sundried tomatoes together. Set aside to soak while you continue. In a food processor, process all the other ingredients together except the fresh herbs. Remove this wet mixture and set aside. Drain the seed mixture and blend in the food processor until well chopped. Add the vegetable mixture to the food processor and pulse all together. Roughly chop the fresh herbs and pulse through the mixture. Roll into balls and flatten into hemp burger patties. Dehydrate for 4–6 hours at 116°F (47°C).

Serve with a fresh salad, slices of tomato, bao-mayo (see page 38) and hemp onion bread (see below).

HEMP ONION BREAD

Makes 18 slices

- *½ C chia seeds, ground*
- *1 C water*
- *3 large red onions*
- *1 C sunflower seeds*
- *½ C hemp seeds*
- *½ C hemp protein powder*
- *¼ C tamari*
- *¼ C olive oil*
- *¼ C hemp oil*
- *½ t salt*

Place the chia in a large mixing bowl. Add the water, work into a paste, and set aside. In a food processor, slice the onions, using the slicing blade. Transfer to the large mixing bowl. Process the sunflower and hemp seeds in the food processor using the S blade and transfer to the mixing bowl. Add the remaining ingredients to the bowl and combine well by hand. Spread the mixture out onto a teflex sheet on a dehydrator tray. Score it to make cutting easier later on. Dehydrate for 16–18 hours in total, removing it from the teflex sheet after 2–3 hours to speed up the drying on both sides.

Take one slice of bread and load it up with your favorite toppings, e.g., bao-mayo, pesto, avocado, tomato, and salad. Top with another slice of bread and cut diagonally to make beautiful and delicious sandwiches.

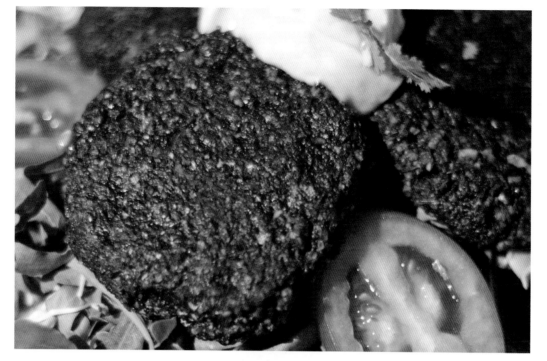

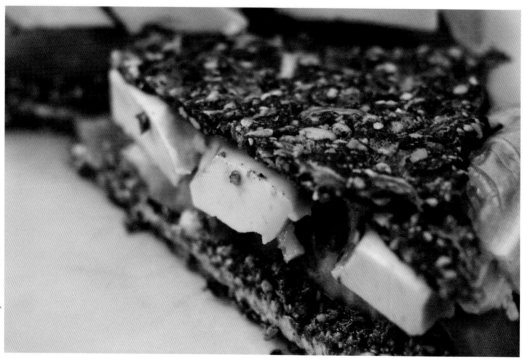

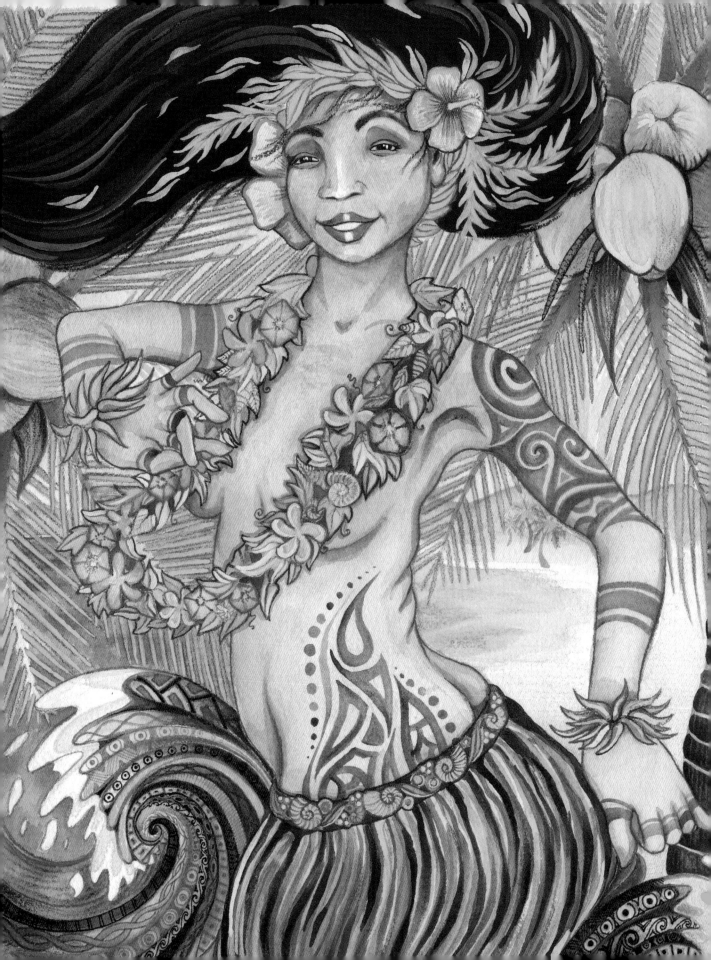

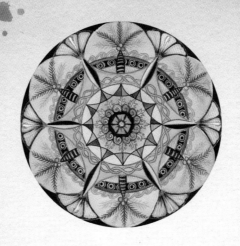

COCONUT

THE TREE THAT SUPPLIES ALL THAT IS NEEDED TO LIVE

REVITALIZING ELECTROLYTES * WEIGHT LOSS

REDUCED CHOLESTEROL * ENERGY BOOSTING * IMMUNE ENHANCING

HORMONE BALANCING * BLOOD SUGAR BALANCING

SKIN HEALTH * REPRODUCTIVE HEALTH * BEST COOKING OIL

Sway to the rhythm, the dance of life,
She moves like the ocean, her body strong and lithe,
Coconut traveling on the sea's undulation
To land on the shore and begin transformation
But even as she becomes a tall palm tree
She will never truly forget the sea:
Coconut water, a fine-tuned composition,
An electrolyte blend that is perfect nutrition.
There's an elemental resonance, a fluid link
'tween the ocean, our blood, and the coconut drink.

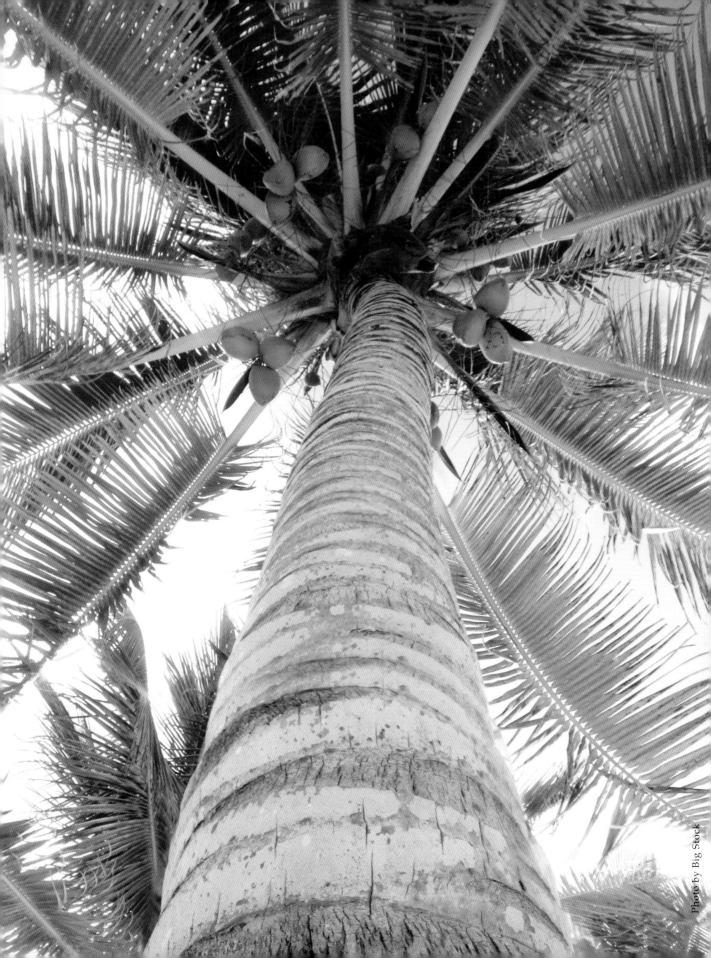

ANCIENT, REVERED SUPERFOOD

The coconut is truly one of nature's most abundant gifts. In Sanskrit, the coconut palm is known as the *kalpa vriksha*, which means "the tree that supplies all that is needed to live." The closest match in nature to mother's milk is found within the coconut. This tropical staple is loaded with many powerful fatty acids that give it its delicious taste and an abundance of health-enhancing benefits.

Coconut palms are prehistoric plants related to grasses, making them extremely salt tolerant and allowing them to grow right next to the ocean. They are able to absorb almost every mineral needed for human nutrition. Coconuts have spread around the tropical regions of the world by their ability to survive for many months afloat at sea. The coconut is a natural water filter, taking almost nine months to filter a liter of water into the shell.

Young coconuts are the most health supportive, providing a delicious soft meat and up to 16 oz of pure coconut water. Older coconuts are used to press out coconut oil, a delicious, creamy, and nutritious fat that is solid and white when cool and clear liquid when warmed. Coconut oil, water, and cream have been used for centuries not only nutritionally but also cosmetically and therapeutically.

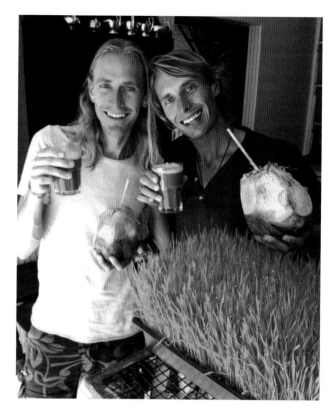

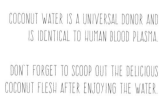

COCONUT WATER IS A UNIVERSAL DONOR AND
IS IDENTICAL TO HUMAN BLOOD PLASMA.

DON'T FORGET TO SCOOP OUT THE DELICIOUS
COCONUT FLESH AFTER ENJOYING THE WATER.

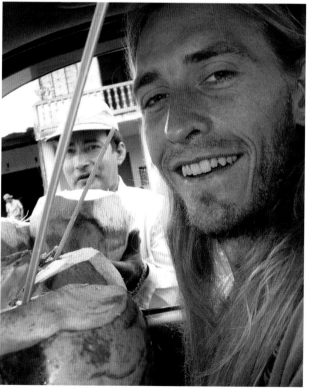

HOW WE USE COCONUT PRODUCTS

There is nothing quite like sitting on a tropical beach sipping the water from a fresh young coconut! Young coconuts are widely available now, so you don't have to go on holiday to have some. Buy them fresh, make sure no mold is visible, and then cut through the green skin at the top to find the "eyes." They are little holes that can be punctured with a pointed knife to get a straw in.

Coconut oil is another way to get the benefits of coconut without having to brandish a weapon. Look for cold-pressed organic brands. Coconut water, meat, and oil can all be used to make superfood drinks and recipes. We like to use the oil to make chocolate sauce and the water to make coconut kefir, a live probiotic drink! Coconut flakes are a great ingredient in muesli and also for making macaroons. Coconut cream is available in tins. Make sure there are no preservatives or other strange ingredients, or make your own by blending the soft meat from the coconut with its water. Coconut sugar is made from coconut blossoms and is a low-GI alternative to toxic refined sugars.

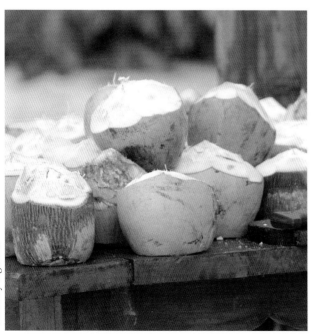

Photo by Big Stock

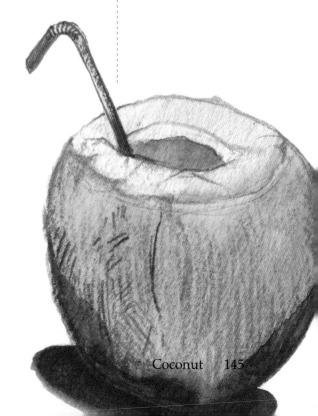

THE MAGIC OF COCONUTS

- REVITALIZING ELECTROLYTES
- WEIGHT LOSS
- REDUCED CHOLESTEROL
- ENERGY BOOSTING
- IMMUNE ENHANCING
- HORMONE BALANCING
- BLOOD SUGAR BALANCING
- SKIN HEALTH
- REPRODUCTIVE HEALTH
- BEST COOKING OIL

Revitalizing electrolytes

Coconut water is one of the highest sources of electrolytes known in nature and is almost identical to human blood plasma, making it a universal donor and great for rehydration. Coconut water was used to give emergency plasma transfusions to wounded soldiers during World War II.

Weight loss

The saturated medium-chain fatty acids (MCFAs) in coconut speeds up the thyroid gland, which speeds up metabolism, allowing the body to drop excess weight and toxins. Coconut cannot be stored in the body as fat, as it is burned up in metabolism immediately.

Reduced cholesterol

Contrary to the common misconception, coconut oil contains no cholesterol, and actually helps to reduce cholesterol levels by converting it into healthy hormones, outperforming even cold-pressed olive oil! Coconut-eating cultures in the tropics have consistently lower cholesterol levels than people in the United States. Coconut oil is a raw saturated fat, containing mostly MCFAs. Coconut supports the formation of healthy HDL cholesterol in the liver. Most information relating to saturated fat is inaccurate. The mass media have led us to believe that saturated fat is bad and causes cholesterol, when in fact it is high-calorie, long-chain saturated animal fat found in meat and dairy and rancid unsaturated fat found in cooked vegetable oils that leads to the clogging of the arteries.

Energy boosting

The MCFAs in coconut oil require less energy and fewer enzymes to digest without burdening the liver and gall bladder. This provides more energy more quickly than other fat sources.

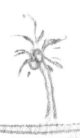

Immune enhancing

The MCFAs in coconut have powerful antiviral, antimicrobial, and antifungal properties. They disrupt the cell membranes of bacteria, viruses, and yeast, allowing the immune system's white blood cells to consume them. The caprylic acid in coconut is one of the most potent yeast-fighting substances, excellent in helping overcome candida infections.

Hormone balancing

Coconut products stimulate the thyroid to release more thyroid hormones, which in turn convert cholesterol in the body into the anti-aging master hormone pregnenalone. Pregnenalone is then converted into progesterone, one of our most important anti-aging hormones.

Blood sugar balancing

Coconut foods are excellent at relieving hunger and causing blood sugar levels to remain stable for longer. Stable blood sugar levels mean relief from the effects of adrenal stress.

Skin health

Coconut oil reverses tissue damage. It has been used as a skin moisturizer for thousands of years. Everyday common lotions provide temporary relief from dry skin, but weaken the skin over time. Coconut oil's antiseptic elements keep the skin healthy and youthful. It also makes the best natural tanning lotion.

Reproductive health

According to Ayurvedic medicine, young coconut meat is the best builder of male sexual fluids of any food. In women, the meat is easily developed into breast milk and is an excellent supportive food during and after pregnancy. Coconut oil is also an excellent personal lubricant!

Best cooking oil

Coconut oil is the most stable of all oils. Therefore, it is the only oil you should ever consider using for your cooking or frying needs. Because it is a completely saturated fat, it does not turn into dangerous trans fats (cancer-forming bad fats) when cooked. All other oils, including butter, margarine, olive oil, canola oil, corn oil, seed oils, and so on, are unstable and can denature when excessive heat is applied!

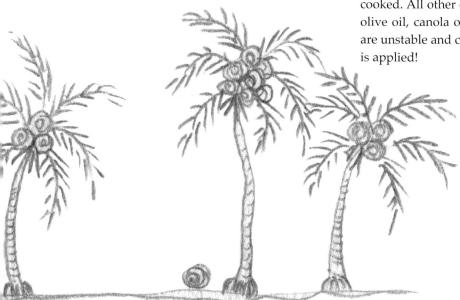

COCONUT RECIPES

—————⟳—————

COCONUT WATER * COCONUT MILK * COCONUT KEFIR

COCONUT-BASED SMOOTHIES * COCONUT, BANANA, AND CHOCOLATE CREPES

COCONUT ICE CREAM CONES * MANGO CUSTARD

MATT`S THAI GREEN COCONUT CURRY

—————⟳—————

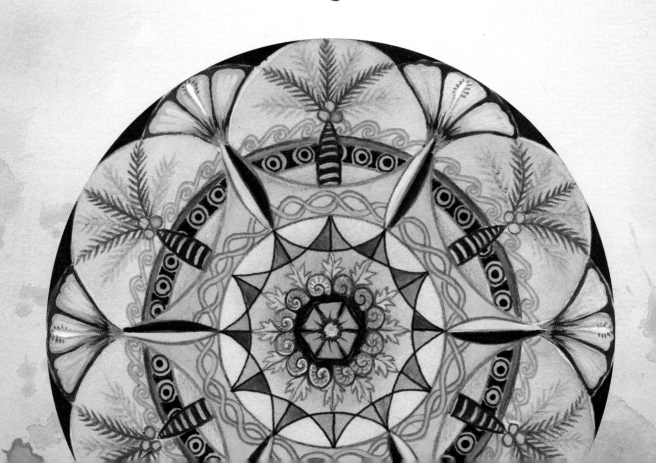

COCONUT WATER

Puncture a hole into the softest of the three holes, or eyes, of a young green or brown coconut. Insert a straw and savor the water that the coconut palm has taken nine months to filter into the most amazing rehydrating liquid of life.

COCONUT MILK

Cut open the coconut and blend the soft inner flesh with water or the coconut water to make your own coconut milk.

COCONUT KEFIR

Coconut kefir is fermented coconut water. You get the benefits of not only the coconut water, but the good bacteria formed during the fermenting process.

Find yourself some water kefir grains. Add them to fresh coconut water and stir. With the lid loosely on, leave out of the fridge to ferment. After twenty-four hours put it in the fridge and enjoy chilled. It gets better as it ages.

Photo by Luke Daniel

COCONUT-BASED SMOOTHIES

Add coconut water, milk, or kefir into your smoothies or replace the water in smoothie recipes with the coconut liquid for enhanced nourishment. You can also add coconut oil to smoothies. One word of caution, though—coconut oil and white mulberries taste strange when blended together, so steer clear of adding coconut oil to any of the mulberry drink recipes.

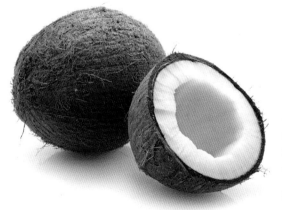

Photo by Big Stock

COCONUT, BANANA, AND CHOCOLATE CREPES

Makes 2 large crepes

> 1 C desiccated coconut, soaked
>   in 1 C of warm water
> 4 bananas
> ½ C flax, ground, or ⅛ C psyl-
>   lium husk powder
> juice of ½ lemon
> ⅛ t salt
> ¼ C raw cacao powder
>   (optional to make chocolate
>   crepes)

Blend all the ingredients together, including the soak water, and spread into a large crepe shape on a teflex sheet. Put into the dehydrator and allow to dry for 2–3 hours. Then flip the crepe off the teflex sheet onto the mesh sheet and allow the other side to dry for another 2–3 hours. Repeat for second crepe.

COCONUT ICE CREAM CONES

Makes 4 cones

Making ice cream cones is so easy. You simply take the recipe for the crepes (above), add one extra step, and carry on drying them.

At the point when you would have eaten them as crepes, while they are still soft and pliable, cut the crepes in half and roll into cone shapes. Then put a small shot glass in the cones to hold them open, and return them to the dryer for approximately 10–12 hours or until crispy.

Scoop your favorite raw ice cream into a cone and enjoy.

MANGO CUSTARD

Makes 2 C

> 2–3 mangoes
> ⅛ C coconut oil, melted

This recipe is in *Rawlicious* as part of the apple tart served with custard, but it's such a delicious custard that it deserves to stand alone. When people taste it, they can't believe it's only two ingredients! When mangoes are in season, make a big batch and keep it in the fridge—it stores beautifully.

Blend the ingredients together in a power blender until smooth and creamy. Serve and enjoy.

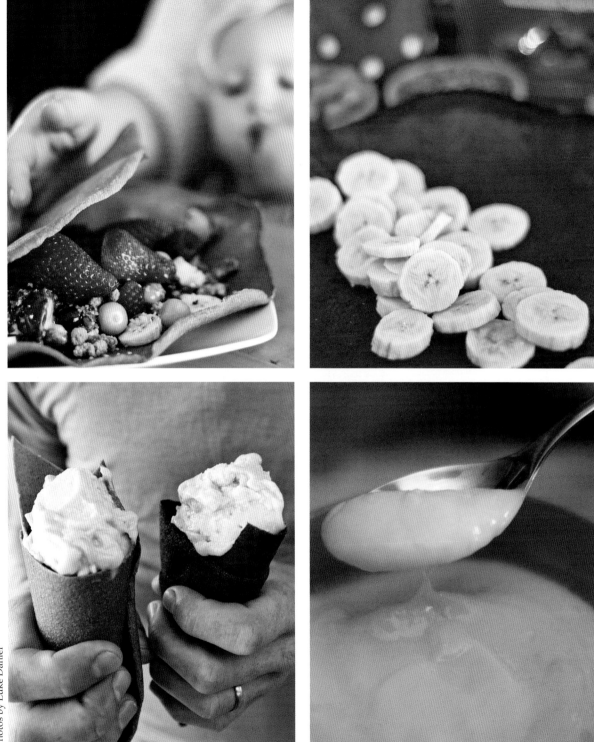

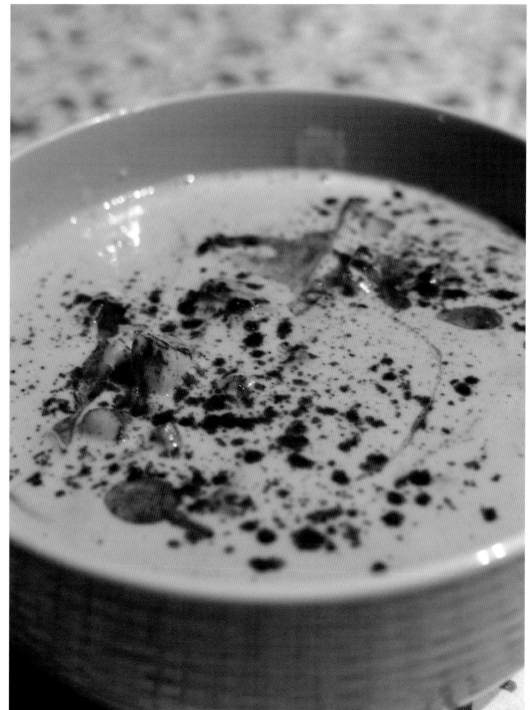

MATT'S THAI GREEN COCONUT CURRY

Matt is a friend of ours who loves to drink his food. He is so in love with his blender that he rigged up his Land Cruiser to be able to power a Vitamix and took his blender with him on a London to Cape Town mega-Africa road trip!

Whenever Matt has us round for dinner, I always ask him to make this dish—it's my favorite.

Blend all the sauce ingredients until smooth. Place the sauce in a pot and warm through. Slice the zucchini using a mandolin to approximately 1 mm thick, and then cut to look like bamboo shoots. Slice other veggies and add to the warm sauce.

Serve in large bowls.

Serves 4

For the sauce:

1 C coconut oil
2 avocados
2 dried lime leaves
¼–½ fresh chili or chili powder
1 t lime or lemon juice
¾ in lemongrass stem
½ in cube of fresh ginger
handful of cashews
½ C loosely packed fresh coriander
½–1 C of water (add more to make it thinner or to suit the amount of vegetables you cut up)
½ T of curry powder (add more to spice it up as you like)
salt to taste
pepper to taste

The vegetables:

zucchini
tender-stem baby broccoli
baby corn
peppers

Other delicious recipes that include desiccated coconut are maca-roons (see page 175) and the goji and orange carrot cake (see page 54).

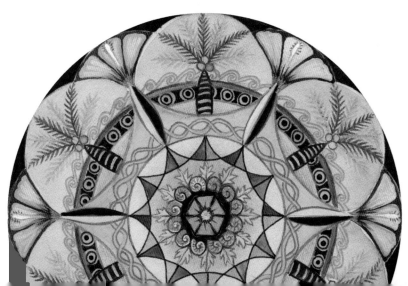

153

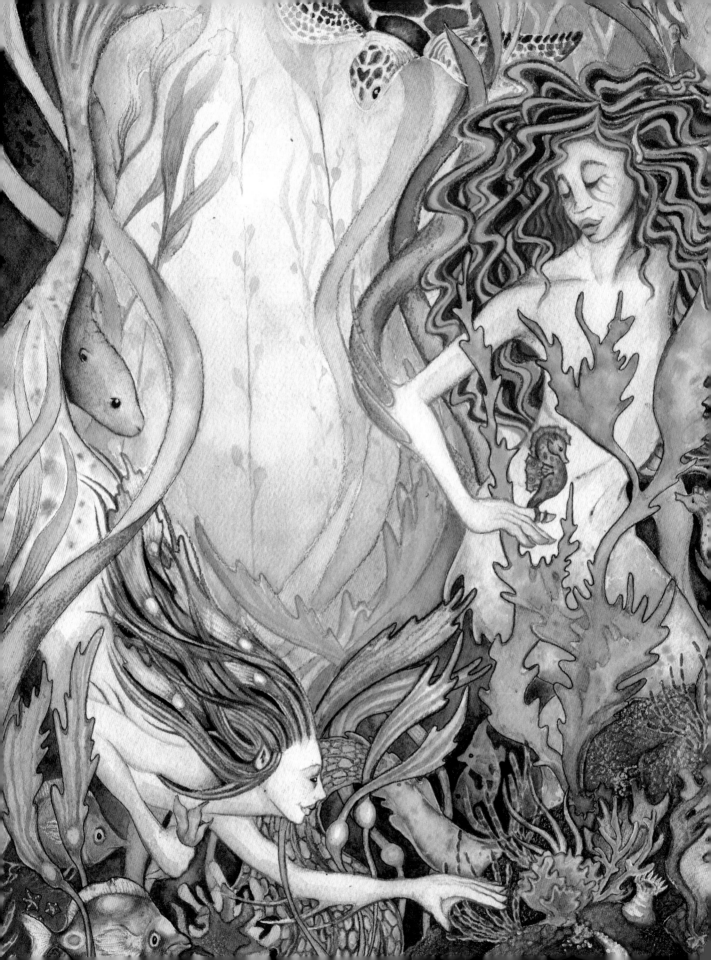

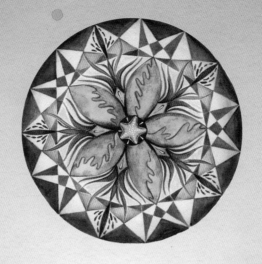

SEA VEGETABLES
WILD MINERAL GIFTS FROM THE SEA

HEALTHY THYROID FUNCTION ✶ CANCER PROTECTION

CARDIOVASCULAR DISEASE PREVENTION ✶ ADRENAL SUPPORT

FOLIC ACID RICH ✶ MINERAL RICH

LONGEVITY ANTIOXIDANTS ✶ HEAVY METAL DETOXIFICATION

Beneath the breakers lies a mysterious world,
Of colors so vivid, tides rhythmically swirled,
Kelp forest, aqua forest, underwater city,
Supporting myriad life forms and rich complexity.
Where mermaids harvest seaweed of various hues,
Wild mineral gifts that a human can use.
The balance in our bodies and in the ocean's connected:
When we take care of the one, the other's affected.
So let us tend both with deep dedication,
And gratefully acknowledge with every inhalation;
After all, life would falter and cease its motion
Without the earth's great circulation pump that is the ocean.

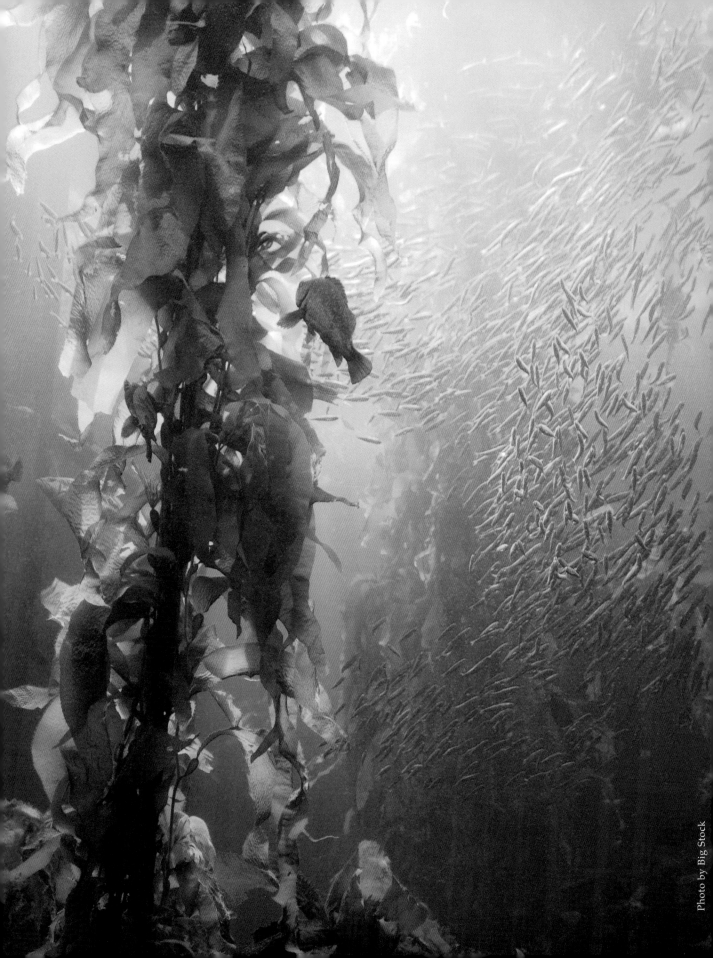

ANCIENT, REVERED SUPERFOOD

Western cultures are only recently beginning to enjoy the taste and nutritional value of sea vegetables, often referred to as seaweed, which have been a staple of the Japanese diet for centuries. The mixture of vitamins, minerals, and trace elements found in seaweeds so closely resembles that of the human body that these healing elements are easily absorbed through the digestive tract into the blood. Some researchers are beginning to believe seaweed alone is an almost perfect solution to many health challenges.

Seaweeds are virtually fat-free, very low in calories, and the richest sources of minerals in the vegetable kingdom. Because they grow in the sea, seaweeds naturally absorb an abundance of the minerals found in the ocean. From decades of over-farming we are facing a shortage of mineral-rich foods because the minerals in the soil are not being replaced. Farmers simply add nitrogen and potassium to the soil to make the plants look good. Instead, we now have to turn to the sea to access the mineral profile that we need from our food in order to thrive.

The sea contains all ninety-two minerals in a balanced proportion identical to that of humans. Sea vegetables contain large amounts of calcium and phosphorus and are extremely high in magnesium, iron, iodine, and sodium.

Seaweed also contains a wide variety of vitamins, including vitamins A, B1, C, and E, concentrated protein, and healthy carbohydrates. It may well be the most nutritionally packed food on the planet. There are thousands of types of sea vegetables. They are classified into categories by color, namely brown, red, or green sea vegetables. Each is unique, having a distinct shape, taste, and texture. Although not all sea vegetables that exist are currently consumed, a wide range of sea vegetables are enjoyed as foods.

SEAWEEDS GROW IN THE DENSEST NUTRIENT SOUP, THE SEA!

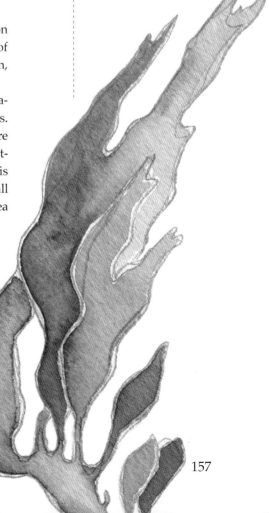

157

The most popular types of sea vegetables are the following:

Nori

Nori has a dark purple-black color that turns phosphorescent green when toasted. It is famous for its role in making sushi rolls. Nori has a sweet, meaty taste when dried. It contains nearly 50% balanced, assimilable protein, more than any other sea plant. Nori is rich in all the carotenes, calcium, iodine, iron, and phosphorus.

Kelp

Kelp is light brown to dark green in color, and is often available in flake or powder form. Kelp grows abundantly on the Western Cape coastline. It contains vitamins A, B, E, D, and K, and is a rich source of vitamin C and minerals. Kelp contains sodium alginate (algin), which helps remove radioactive particles and heavy metals from the body. Algin, carrageenan, and ager are kelp gels that rejuvenate gastrointestinal health and aid digestion. Kelp works as a blood purifier, relieves arthritis and stiffness, and promotes adrenal, pituitary, and thyroid health. Kelp's natural iodine can normalize thyroid-related disorders such as obesity and lymph system congestion.

Hijiki

This sea vegetable looks like small strands of black wiry pasta and has a strong flavor. Hijiki is a mineral-rich, high-fiber seaweed, with 20% protein, vitamin A, carotenes, and calcium. Hijiki has the most calcium of any sea vegetable: 1,400 mg per 100 g of dry weight.

Kombu

Kombu is very dark in color and is generally sold in strips or sheets. It is often used as a flavoring for soups. Kombu has a long tradition as a Japanese delicacy with great nutritional healing value. It is a decongestant for excess mucus and helps normalize blood pressure. Kombu has abundant iodine, carotenes, vitamins B, C, D, and E, minerals such as calcium, magnesium, potassium, silica, iron, and zinc, and the powerful skin-healing nutrient germanium. Kombu is a meaty, high-protein seaweed. It is higher in natural mineral salts than most other seaweeds.

Wakame

Similar to kombu, wakame is most commonly used to make Japanese miso soup. Wakame is a high-protein, high-calcium seaweed, with carotenes, iron, and vitamin C.

Arame

This lacy, wiry sea vegetable is sweeter and milder in taste than many others. Arame is one of the ocean's richest sources of iodine. Herbalists use arame to help reduce breast and uterine fibroids and, through its fat-soluble vitamins and phytohormones, to normalize menopausal symptoms. Arame promotes soft, wrinkle-free skin, enhances glossy hair, and prevents hair loss.

Dulse

With a soft, chewy texture and a reddish-brown color, dulse is our favorite mineral snack! Dulse is rich in iron, protein, and vitamin A. It is a supremely balanced food, with three hundred times more iodine and fifty times more iron than wheat. Tests on dulse show activity against the herpes virus. It has purifying and tonic effects on the body.

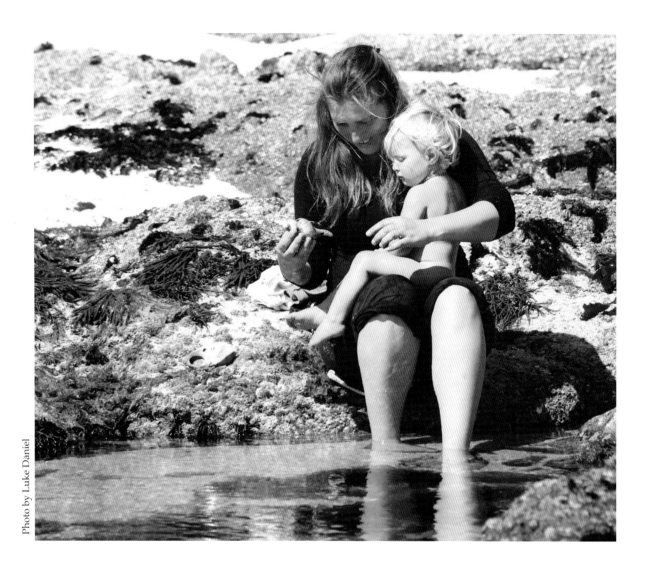

Photo by Luke Daniel

Sea lettuce

Sea lettuce is the "salad greens" of sea vegetables. It is a leafy, vibrant dark green, with a delicious, delicate flavor. This sea vegetable is best raw, and is good in soups or salads. Experiment by tearing or cutting the whole dry leaves with scissors into your favorite dish. Nutritionally it is very high in dietary fiber, iron, and protein (similar to dulse), and high in iodine, manganese, and nickel.

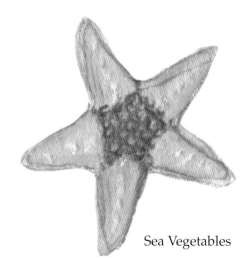

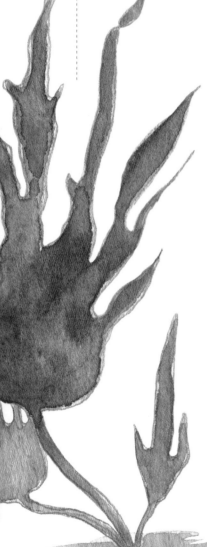

LIKE TREES IN A FOREST, KELP PLANTS PROVIDE SHELTER AND HABITAT FOR AN ENORMOUS NUMBER AND DIVERSITY OF ANIMALS, INCLUDING FISH, SEA SNAILS, AND CRABS.

SEA VEGETABLES ARE A GREAT SOURCE OF MINERALS, AS THE SEA CONTAINS ALL KNOWN MINERALS.

THE MAGIC OF SEA VEGETABLES

HEALTHY THYROID FUNCTION

CANCER PROTECTION

CARDIOVASCULAR DISEASE PREVENTION

ADRENAL SUPPORT

FOLIC ACID RICH

MINERAL RICH

LONGEVITY ANTIOXIDANTS

HEAVY METAL DETOXIFICATION

Healthy thyroid function

Seaweed is nature's richest source of iodine, a component of the thyroid hormones, which are essential to human life. The thyroid gland adds iodine to the amino acid tyrosine to create these hormones. Without sufficient iodine, your body cannot synthesize them. Because these thyroid hormones regulate metabolism in every cell of the body and play a role in virtually all physiological functions, an iodine deficiency can have a devastating impact on your health and well-being. Kelp is a particularly excellent source of iodine.

Cancer protection

Lignans inhibit angiogenesis, or blood cell growth, the process through which fast-growing tumors send cancer cells into the bloodstream to establish secondary tumors in other areas of the body. Lignans, found in sea vegetables, also inhibit estrogen synthesis in fat cells. High levels of certain estrogen metabolites are considered a significant risk factor for breast cancer. Seaweed is a very good source of the B vitamin folic acid. Studies have shown that diets high in folate-rich foods are associated with a significantly reduced risk for colon cancer.

Cardiovascular disease prevention

Sea vegetables protect against heart disease. They are a very good source of magnesium, which reduces high blood pressure and helps to prevent heart attacks.

Adrenal support

Two B vitamins—pantothenic acid and riboflavin—are necessary for energy production. Pantothenic acid is especially important for the health of the adrenal glands. Stressful times can exhaust the adrenal glands, resulting in chronic fatigue, reduced resistance to allergies and infection, and a feeling of being overwhelmed or overly anxious. These B vitamins are readily available in sea vegetables.

Folic acid rich

Studies have shown that adequate levels of folic acid in the diet are needed to prevent certain birth defects, including spina bifida. Folic acid is also needed to break down dangerous homocysteine levels. Homocysteine can directly damage blood vessel walls, and high levels are associated with a significantly increased risk of cardiovascular disease and stroke.

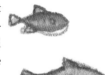

Mineral rich

Sea vegetables offer your body ten to twenty times the minerals of land plants. Because they grow in the sea, seaweeds naturally absorb an abundance of the minerals found in the ocean.

Longevity antioxidants

A well-studied brown kelp variety, *Ecklonia cava,* contains compounds that are currently being hailed as super-antioxidants. One such compound, eckol, has been shown to protect lung cells from oxidative damage. Another compound found in *Ecklonia cava* is potent polyphenols. Polyphenols have antioxidant properties and multiple health benefits. Studies have shown remarkable results treating conditions such as fibromyalgia, high cholesterol, hypertension, diabetes, allergies, asthma, arthritis, and neuropathy.

Heavy metal detoxification

Alginic acid is a polysaccharide that is abundant in sea vegetables. Research demonstrates that alginic acid binds with any heavy metals found in the intestines, renders them indigestible, and causes them to be eliminated. Any heavy metals—such as barium, cadmium, lead, mercury, and even radioactive strontium, which may be present in the intestines—will not be absorbed by the body when alginic acid is present.

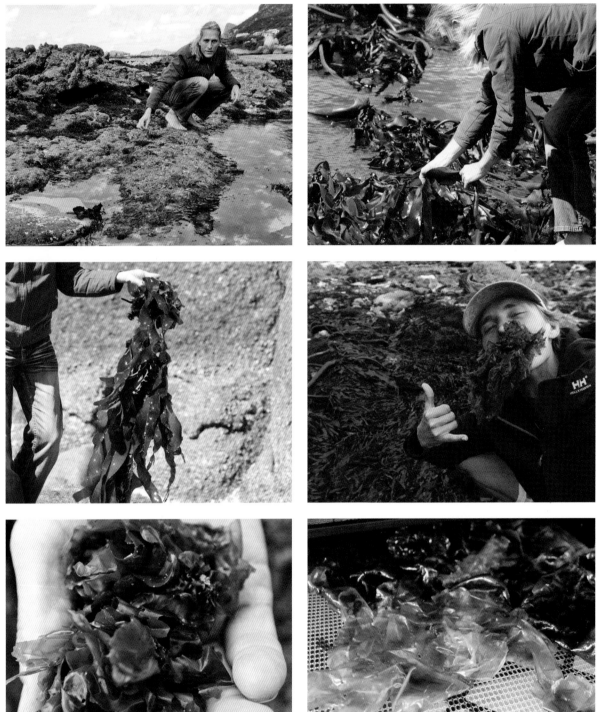

Photos by Luke Daniel

HOW WE USE SEA VEGETABLES

We regularly go on wild food outings to forage for our own sea vegetables. We collect the seaweeds at low tide, making sure to be as far as possible from built-up areas to avoid pollution. We then wash them in freshwater and dehydrate them for up to twelve hours. Once dry, they are easily powdered in a blender to make a jar of superpotent seaweed powder.

Nori: Sold as sushi sheets. Great to make hand rolls.

Arame: Soak for five minutes and add raw to salad, rice, or freshly chopped veggies. Good with a vinaigrette dressing.

Dulse: Does not require cooking. Try using dulse flakes as a condiment. It is easily sprinkled on top of soups, salads, and veggies. Slightly salty and smoky in flavor, it is a nutritious alternative to salt for those on low- or no-salt diets.

Hijiki: Rinse, then soak for twenty minutes and rinse again. It expands over four times when soaked. It tastes great flavored with sesame oil, cider vinegar, and tamari.

Kelp: Use as a salt substitute or condiment in powder form. It acts as a natural tenderizer when added to beans and stews.

Kombu: Best used in slow-cooking soups, beans, and stews to both flavor and tenderize. Add a whole piece about two to four inches long, remove once tender, chop up, and place back in the dish.

Wakame: Soak for five minutes before using, then rinse; or add directly to soups without soaking. This is the seaweed most often added to miso soup. With its sweet flavor, it also makes a great cold salad.

Sea lettuce: Looks just like lettuce! Despite a strong seafood taste and odor, it's delicate after drying and crumbles easily into tiny, tender pieces. Blend up a variety of sea vegetables in a power blender to make a sea vegetable powder mix that can be added to soups, salads, and sauces.

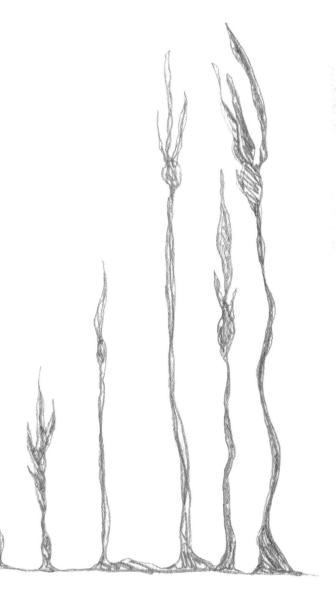

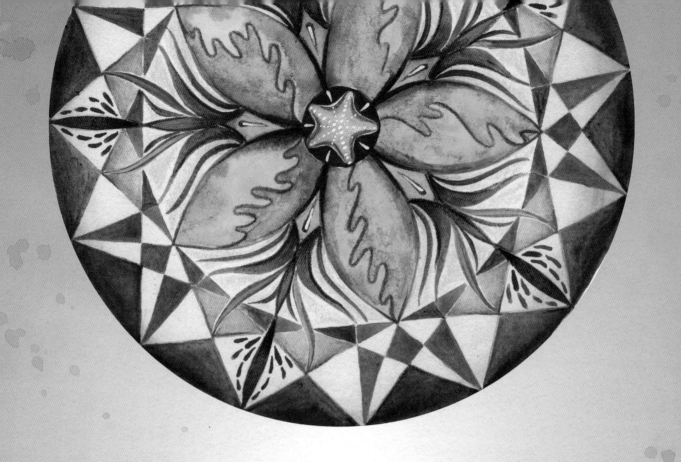

SEA VEGETABLE RECIPES

SUSHI HANDROLLS ✶ MERMAID SOUP ✶ KELP NOODLES
NORI WANDS ✶ SEA VEG GUACAMOLE ✶ SEAWEED SALAD
CUCUMBER, AVOCADO, AND DULSE BITES

SUSHI HANDROLLS

raw nori sheets
parsnip, turnip, or cauliflower rice
  (see below for details)
avocado slices
carrots, julienned
cucumber, julienned
red pepper, julienned
a selection of sprouts
rocket leaves
wasabi
ginger
tamari

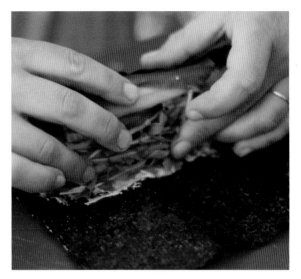

Parsnip rice

Our favorite rice for making sushi handrolls is parsnip rice—it is sweet and delicious. You can substitute the parsnips for turnips or a small head of cauliflower instead.

4 parsnips, peeled
2 garlic cloves
1 T olive oil
½ t salt
juice of 1 lemon
½ T tamari sauce

In a food processor, process the parsnips until well chopped, resembling a rice consistency. Add the other ingredients to flavor and pulse through.

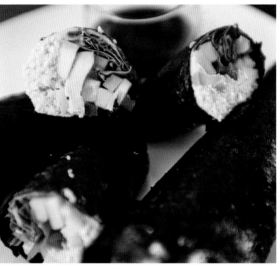

Assembling a handroll

Place a raw nori sheet on a chopping board. Place a layer of rice on the bottom half of the nori sheet. Layer the avocado, carrots, cucumber, and red pepper. Top with the sprouts and rocket leaves, and roll into a handroll by tucking in both ends, rolling, and slicing in half. Serve with wasabi, ginger, and tamari.

Tips:

Pickle your own ginger by finely slicing ginger and adding it to apple cider vinegar with a touch of beetroot juice for 24 hours or longer.

You can get wasabi powder that just requires you to add water and that does not contain strange E-number additives, which a lot of the wasabi tubes contain.

MERMAID SOUP

Sea vegetables can be described as the last bastion of original food. They haven't been tampered with or altered by cross-breeding or genetic modification. They are a true heirloom food source that is packed with trace minerals. The sea contains all ninety-two minerals needed for real nutrition, and the plants that grow in the sea have access to all of them.

Another one of Katara's favorites, this is an excellent way to get all the nutritional benefits of sea vegetables and algae into you and your children.

Makes 1.5 qt

> *1 qt hot water*
> *1 T miso*
> *1 avocado*
> *¼ onion*
> *⅓ in ginger*
> *1 garlic clove*
> *3 T seaweed powder mix (a dulse, sea lettuce, and kelp mix or your own)*
> *1 T lemon juice*
> *1 T olive oil*
> *1 T tamari*
> *½ T herbamare*
> *1 t salt*
> *½ t spirulina powder*
> *½ t kelp powder*
> *½ t honey*
> *2 nori sheets*

In a blender, blend all the ingredients together except the nori. Cut the nori into fine strips and stir into the soup. You could also add arame, hijiki, or dulse in at the end.

KELP NOODLES

Kelp noodles take life back to a "two-minute noodle" sense of convenience. You can get clear or green kelp noodles. We love the clear ones because they look so much like pasta noodles.

Serves 2

> *12 oz packet of kelp noodles*

Empty noodles into a bowl and pour warm water over them. Allow to stand for 5–10 minutes while you make the sauce. Drain the noodles and mix with your favorite sauce. Add marinated and dehydrated mushrooms and onions or other diced veggies of your choosing. Serve with a fresh salad or on a bed of finely sliced spinach.

Creamy garlic version

Make up a portion of hemp garlic white sauce (see page 133) and add to the noodles.

Pesto version

Make up a portion of 3-algae hemp and coriander pesto (see page 100) and add to the noodles.

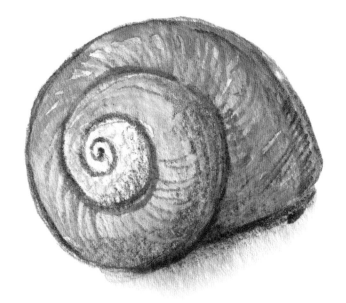

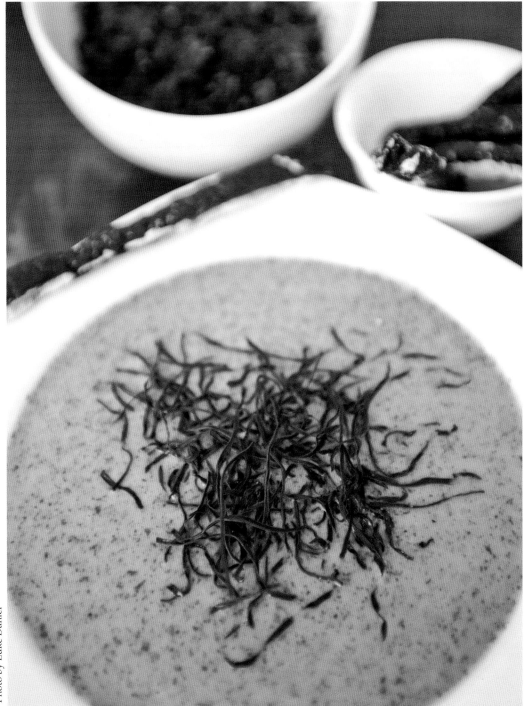

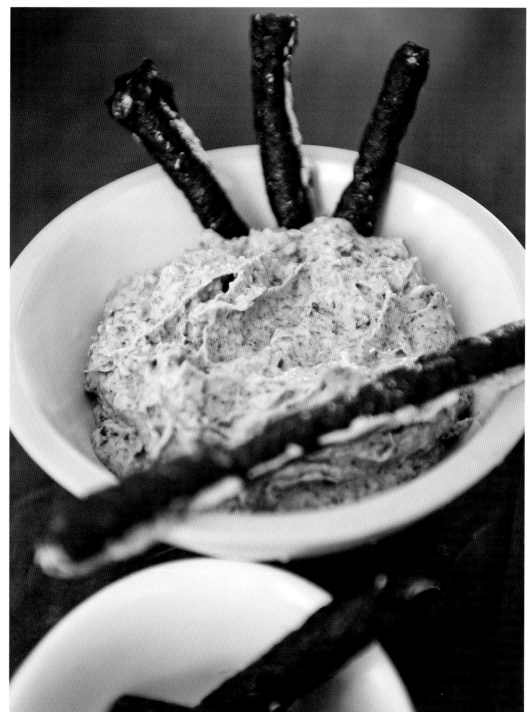

Photo by Luke Daniel

NORI WANDS

These are so tasty—give them a try!

Makes 30 wands

> *10 nori sheets*
> *1 portion of hemp cheese (see page 132)*
> *spring onions, finely sliced*

Take a nori sheet and spread with a thin layer of hemp cheese. Top with spring onions and tightly roll the nori sheet over two or three times to form a thin "wand." Slice it off and keep rolling out the next one. I normally get three wands out of one sheet. Dehydrate for 3–4 hours. *So yum!*

SEAWEED SALAD

This salad is more of a side or accompaniment to a main course salad, but adding it will increase the nutrient density of your meal by miles.

Serves 2

> *1.75 oz (50 g) bag of wakame (presoaked for at least 30 minutes to soften)*
> *2 T tamari sauce*
> *1 T honey*
> *1 T lemon juice*
> *1 T olive oil*
> *1 small clove garlic, finely chopped*
> *¾ in piece ginger, finely chopped*
> *2 T seaweed powder mix*

Drain the wakame and chop into bite-sized pieces (or pulse in a food processor). Place in a bowl and mix through with the other ingredients. It can be eaten straight away, but the flavors will infuse best if you allow it to marinate for about 30 minutes.

SEA VEG GUACAMOLE

We love guacamole, and this takes the nutrient value of guacamole through the roof!

Serves 2–3

> *2 avocados*
> *1 tomato*
> *1 T olive oil*
> *1 garlic clove*
> *¼ red onion*
> *½ t kelp powder*
> *¼ t salt*
> *¼ C water*
> *juice of 1 lemon*
> *1 nori sheet*
> *1 T seaweed powder mix*

Place all the ingredients together in a food processor or power blender and blend until well combined.

CUCUMBER, AVOCADO, AND DULSE BITES

Dulse is a salty, paper-thin seaweed snack that can be eaten exactly as is—straight out of the bag! The flavor combination of this recipe combines salty (dulse), fatty (avocado), and fresh (cucumber) and takes just minutes to prepare.

> *cucumber, sliced into rounds*
> *avocado, diced*
> *dulse strips*

Place the cucumber rounds on a plate, top with a square of avocado, and cover with a slither of dulse on top. Makes as many as desired.

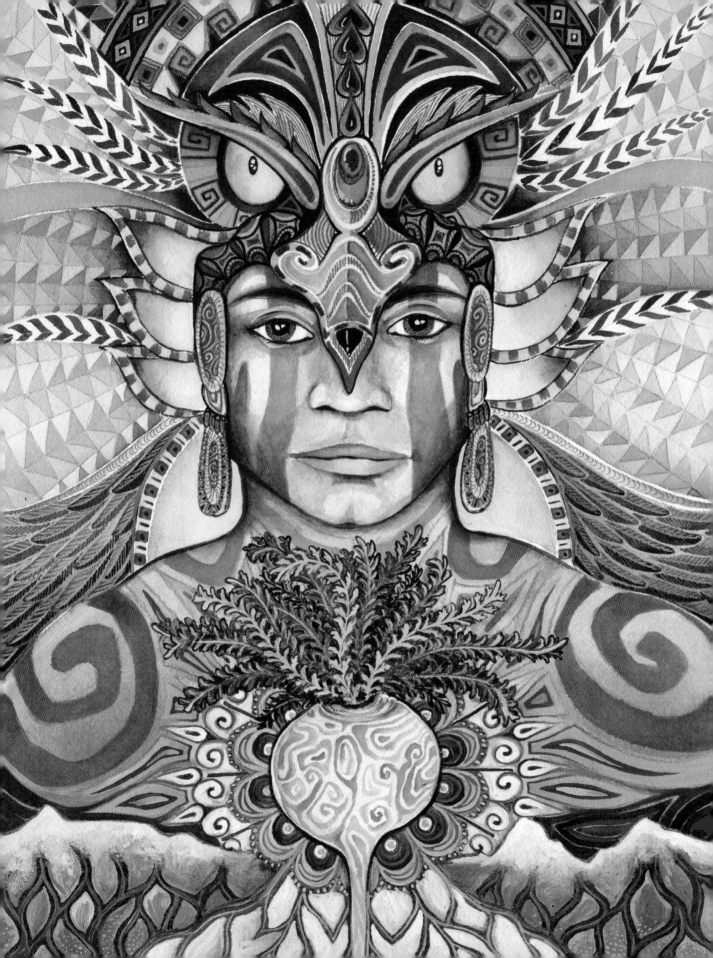

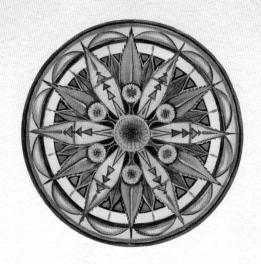

MACA

THE POWER FOOD OF WARRIORS!

⋅⊁╢━━━━━━━━━━━━━━━━━━━╟⊰⋅

IMMUNE SYSTEM SUPPORT ⋅ IMPROVED BRAIN FUNCTION

STRESS SUPPORT ⋅ HORMONAL SUPPORT ⋅ THYROID SUPPORT

NATURE'S APHRODISIAC ⋅ ENHANCED FERTILITY

ATHLETIC SUPPORT ⋅ LONGEVITY

⋅⊁╢━━━━━━━━━━━━━━━━━━━╟⊰⋅

Where the earth's high places meet the sun and the sky
In a mountainous landscape that seems inhospitable and dry
Grows a tuberous root that's become known and acclaimed
For being the Power Food of Warriors, as it is named!
Maca in the ground, a nugget of gold,
A marriage of elements awesome to behold:
Radiant sunlight, earth steady and stable
A body tuned in, strong, responsive, and able.
Energy and stamina, deep steady eyes,
Soaring free as an eagle in cerulean skies.
Endocrine balance, able to change,
In tune with your body, molecules rearrange,
So in every living rhythm, every gesture, every pace,
You may adapt with power, fluidity, and grace.

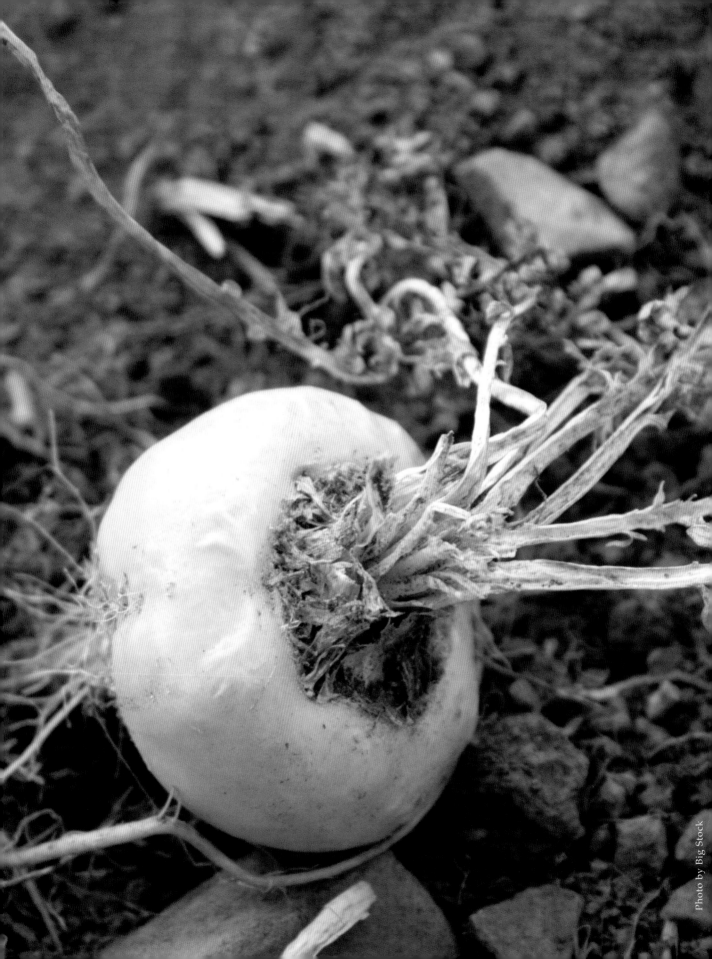

ANCIENT, REVERED SUPERFOOD

Maca is the highest-altitude food-herb grown in the world! Legend has it that Incan warriors used to eat maca before going into battle—they believed it gave them invincible strength and stamina. And truth be told, it probably did!

Like all great superfoods, maca was traded by the ancients and used as money. For centuries (about 2,600 years), the root herb maca has been grown high in the Peruvian Andes mountains, typically at altitudes of over 3,000 meters (9,842 feet) and up to as high as 4,300 meters (14,107 feet). The soils of these high plateaus are extremely rich in minerals, which accounts for maca's amazing array of proteins, trace minerals, and correlating health benefits.

Maca is a cruciferous vegetable similar to a radish. It is exposed to intense levels of sunlight and extreme cold weather conditions. Its ability to survive and thrive against all odds captures its character, and in turn gives you a better ability to adapt to life's myriad of stressors. It is extremely beneficial for people living in cold climates, at high altitudes, and with extreme lifestyles.

Extremely nutrient dense, maca is packed with vitamins, especially vitamins B1, B2, C, and E. It is rich in minerals, including calcium, magnesium, phosphorous, potassium, sulfur, and iron, and contains trace minerals, including zinc, iodine, copper, selenium, bismuth, manganese, and silica. It is a near-complete protein, containing twenty amino acids, seven essential amino acids, and nearly sixty phytochemicals.

MACA IS THE HIGHEST-ALTITUDE CROP IN THE WORLD, GROWING AT AROUND 9,800 FEET ABOVE SEA LEVEL IN THE ANDES.

THE COLOR OF MACA ROOT VARIES FROM CREAMY YELLOW TO RED TO DARK PURPLE OR BLACK.

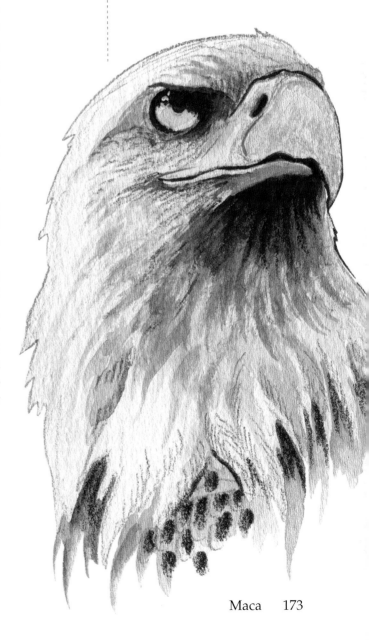

HOW WE USE MACA

Maca tastes malty, like Ovaltine! When we add it to our smoothies, we notice that it not only satisfies the appetite for longer but also gives us more energy and focus. Its simplest application is to add it to smoothies. It is also a great addition to desserts and sweet treats. Maca has an incredible synergistic effect when combined with raw cacao.

You can consume 1–8 t per day to begin with. The more maca you consume, the more benefit you are likely to get. In toxicity studies conducted in the United States, maca showed absolutely no toxicity and no adverse pharmacologic effects

THE MAGIC OF MACA

- IMMUNE SYSTEM SUPPORT
- IMPROVED BRAIN FUNCTION
- STRESS SUPPORT
- HORMONAL SUPPORT
- THYROID SUPPORT
- NATURE'S APHRODISIAC
- ENHANCED FERTILITY
- ATHLETIC SUPPORT
- LONGEVITY

Immune system support

Maca is an adaptogen. Adaptogens boost immunity and increase the body's overall vitality by 10–15% according to most studies.

Improved brain function

Maca increases oxygen levels in the blood, which improves brain function, memory, and mental clarity.

Stress support

As an adaptogen, maca helps your body's metabolism to adapt to stressors, working with your body for optimal results. It has the ability to balance and stabilize the body's systems, helping to increase energy when needed or to calm the system when over-stimulated.

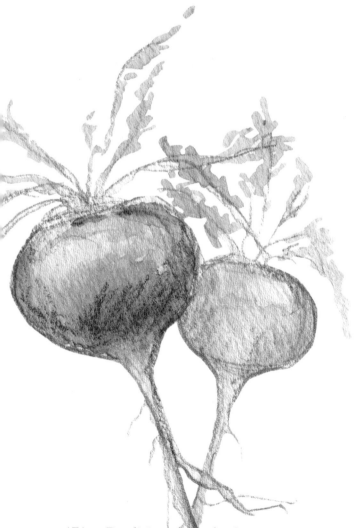

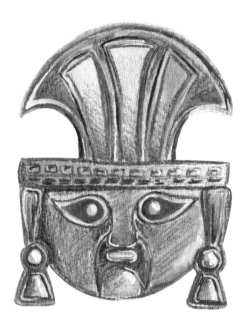

MACA IS WELL-KNOWN FOR PROVIDING RELIEF FROM MENOPAUSAL SYMPTOMS.

THE COLOR OF MACA ROOT VARIES FROM CREAMY YELLOW TO RED TO DARK PURPLE OR BLACK.

Hormonal support

Maca is a great source of hormonal precursors. It stimulates hormone levels by working on the master gland of the brain, the hypothalamus, considered the sex hormone center of the brain. The pituitary gland then secretes LTH and FSH, and the adrenals and gonads are stimulated to secrete testosterone, progesterone, and DHEA.

MALE HORMONE TONIC

According to Dr. Christiane Northrup, maca can help men who struggle with erectile dysfunction, as it stimulates the body to secrete more testosterone.

FEMALE HORMONE TONIC

Women who take maca report less fatigue and greater energy. It can help to regulate and normalize the menstrual cycle, reducing premenstrual tension. Maca also helps women produce more breast milk. It is used as a natural alternative to hormone replacement therapy, providing relief from menopausal symptoms such as hot flashes and night sweats.

Thyroid support

It is widely reported that maca can eliminate thyroid problems. It seems to do so by altering the endocrine system, thus improving thyroid function without directly changing the chemistry of the thyroid.

Nature's aphrodisiac

In both men and women, maca is known as a natural aphrodisiac. Maca increases oxygen levels in the blood, increasing libido. The aromatic isothiocynates in maca have reputed aphrodisiac properties.

Enhanced fertility

Maca has been used for centuries in the Andes to enhance fertility in humans and animals. Its oxygen-increasing, stress-reducing, libido-enhancing qualities combined with overall hormonal support, have gained it a strong reputation as a sexual tonic.

Athletic support

Maca's dense nutritional profile in terms of proteins and minerals, adaptogenic qualities, hormonal support, and its ability to increase blood oxygenation make it an excellent food for athletes, taking ordinary energy, endurance, and strength to peak performance status.

Longevity

As we age, the hormone content of our bodies decreases. Those with a high production of testosterone and/or progesterone are known to stay younger for longer.

MACA RECIPES

MACA-ROONS * MACA LOVE * MACA AND CACAO SMOOTHIE
GREEN PROTEIN BRAIN-POWER SMOOTHIE * MAPLE AND MACA ICE CREAM
STRAWBERRY MACA PASSION * ICED MACAO * MACA OVALTINE * MACA HOT CHOCOLATE

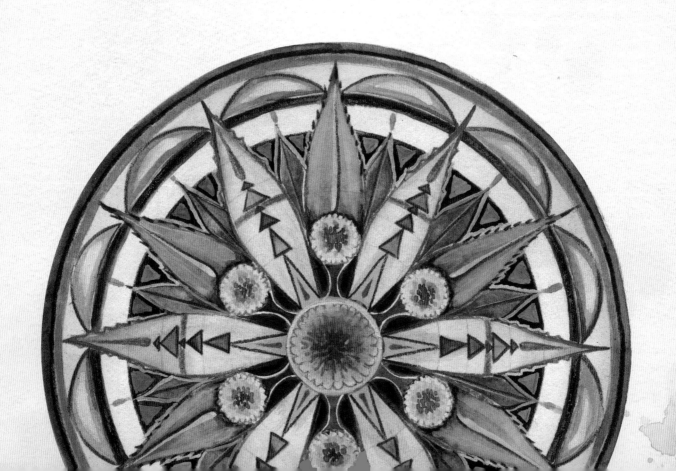

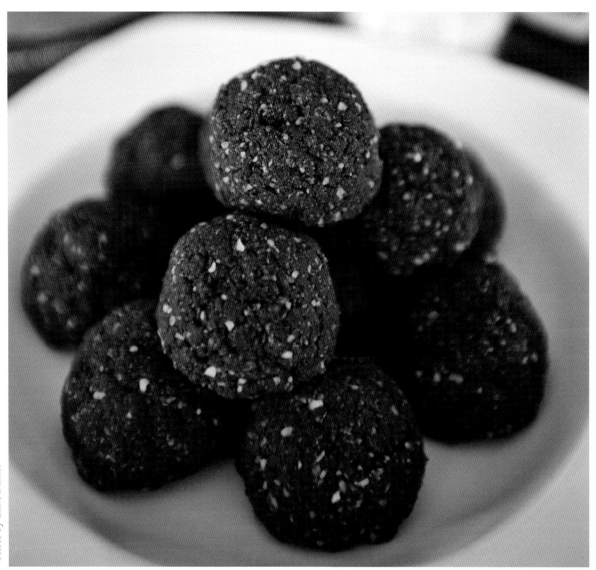

Photo by Luke Daniel

MACA-ROONS

Place all the ingredients together in a food processor and process into a dough-like consistency. Shape into rounds and dehydrate for 6–10 hours. They taste nice after 6 hours, but if you can stop yourself from raiding the dehydrator, they taste even better after 10 hours—they get crispy on the outside and crumbly on the inside!

Makes 15 maca-roons

2 C desiccated coconut
½ C Brazil nuts
½ C maple syrup
¼ C maca
¼ C cacao powder
¼ C cacao butter, melted
1 t vanilla
1 pinch salt

Maca Recipes   177

MACA LOVE

This version of our maca love recipe has become a much-loved favorite in our Rawlicious smoothie bar.

Makes 1 qt

> 2 C water plus ice cubes
> 1½ bananas, frozen
> 1½ T maca
> ¾ C cashews
> 6 dates
> a pinch salt
> ½ t vanilla extract, powder or pod (optional)

Blend all the ingredients together in a blender.

MACA AND CACAO SMOOTHIE

Makes 3 C

> 2 C water
> 1 banana
> ½ C dates
> 2 T maca
> 2 T cacao powder
> 2 T hemp seeds
> ⅛ C Brazil nuts
> ½ t vanilla powder, extract or pod

Blend all the ingredients together in a blender.

GREEN PROTEIN BRAIN-POWER SMOOTHIE

Makes 3 C

> 2 C water
> 1 C ice
> 1 banana (use frozen for extra creaminess)
> 2 T hemp seeds
> 2 T brown rice protein powder
> 2 T pea protein
> 1 T maca
> 1 T chia
> 6 dates
> ½ t spirulina powder
> 1 t wheatgrass powder
> 2 T coconut oil
> ½ t vanilla powder, extract, or pod

Blend all the ingredients together and power up with this mega-protein, green brain-food drink.

MAPLE AND MACA ICE CREAM

This is the maca love smoothie recipe with extra maple syrup stirred through and frozen, so make a double batch of smoothie and freeze half.

Makes 1 qt

> Maca love recipe (see above)
> ⅛ C maple syrup

Make up a jug of the maca love smoothie recipe. Pour into a container and stir in the maple syrup. Freeze.

Tip: The best way to make fluffy ice cream is for the ice cream to be stirred as it is freezing. Using a home ice cream maker makes this easy, but the machine is pricey. Alternatively, stir the mixture through a couple of times by hand during the freezing process. Or, once frozen, press through an Oscar juicer with the solid plate to remove any ice crystals.

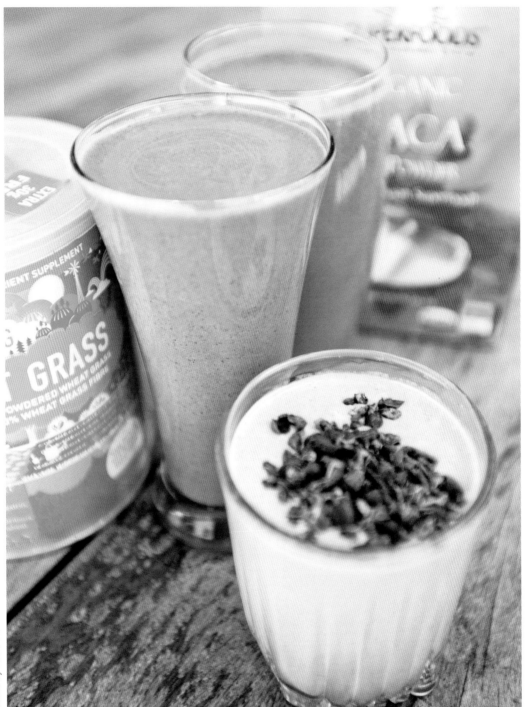

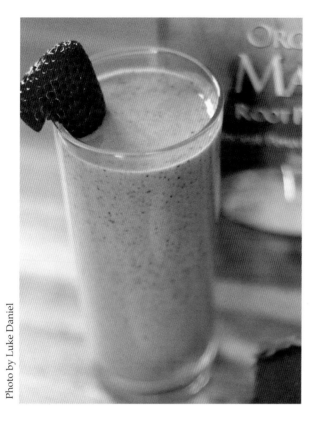

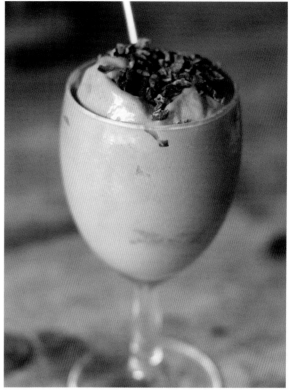

Photo by Luke Daniel

STRAWBERRY MACA PASSION

There is nothing quite like fresh seasonal organic strawberries to ignite the senses. We combined them here with maca for extra passion.

Makes 3 C

> 1 C water
> 1 C strawberries
> 1 banana
> 2 passion fruits
> 1 T maca
> 1 T hemp seeds
> 1 T chia seeds
> 1 T honey

Blend all ingredients together.

ICED MACAO

This drink has a dark, chocolaty flavor. The foti, cacao, and mucuna provide a brain-expanding, stress-reducing effect.

Makes 2 C

> ½ C water
> ½ C cashews
> ⅛ C maple syrup
> 1 T maca
> 1 T foti
> ¼ C cacao powder
> ¼ t mucuna
> 2 C ice
> *cacao nibs (optional)*

First blend all the ingredients, except the ice, until smooth. Lastly, add the ice and blend. You should get a thick icy-textured drink that you can eat with a spoon. Sprinkle with cacao nibs.

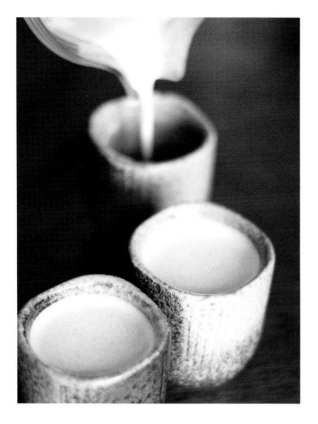

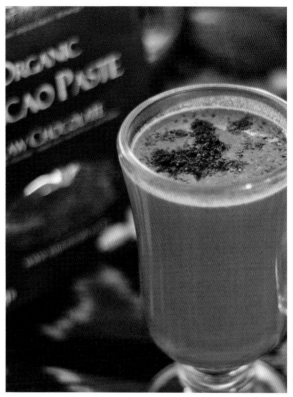

MACA OVALTINE

Maca has a malty flavor, which is delicious as a warm evening drink.

Serves 2

> 2 C hot water
> ¼ C cashews or hemp seeds
> 1½ T maca
> ¼ t vanilla extract
> 1½ T cacao butter
> 1 T lucuma powder
> 2 T honey
> a pinch of salt

Blend and enjoy.

MACA HOT CHOCOLATE

Serves 2

> 1½ C hot water
> 2 T cacao powder
> 1 T maca
> 1 t hemp seeds
> 1 t lucuma powder
> 1 t mesquite
> 2 T honey
> 1 T coconut oil

Blend all the ingredients together and serve.

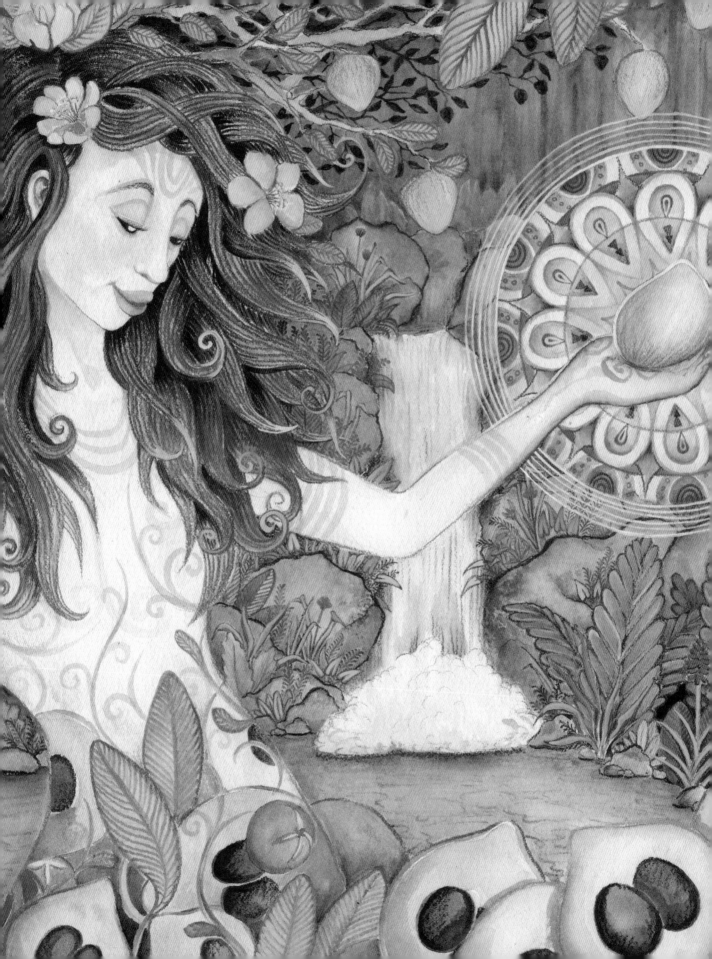

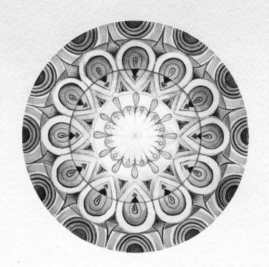

LUCUMA

CREAMY PERUVIAN SUPERFRUIT

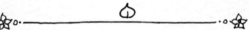

NUTRIENT RICH

LOW-GI SWEETENER

IMMUNE ENHANCING · INCREASED ENERGY

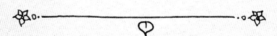

Down by the river near a waterfall,
In the motley shade where the quetzals call,
With gentle hands and flowers in her hair,
She picks the lucuma fruits that grow there.
Creamy and rich, golden and delicious,
Full of energy and highly nutritious,
Your powdery flesh with a butterscotch taste,
A malty sensation, sweetness embraced.
Lady Lucuma with your fruit of gold,
Your harvest is truly a gift to behold.

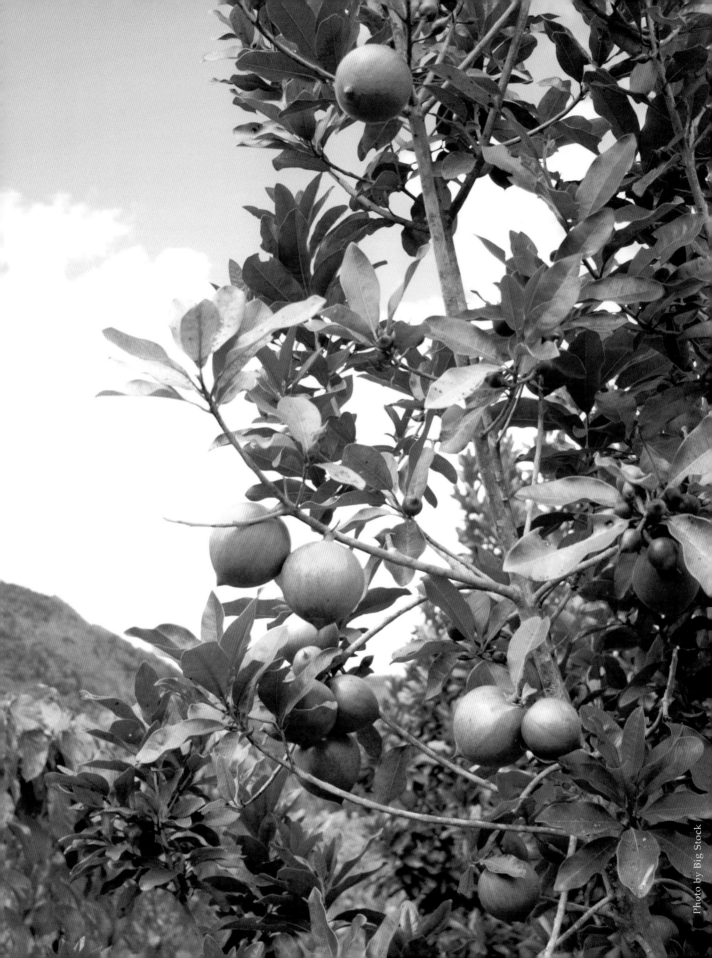

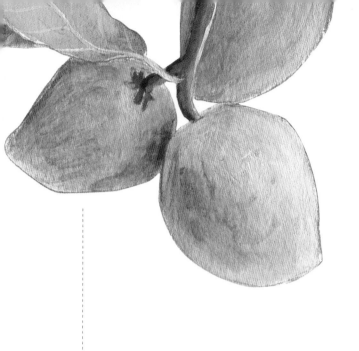

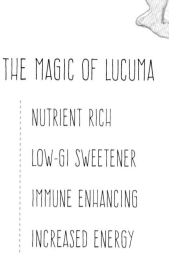

FRESH LUCUMA FRUIT LOOKS JUICY, BUT IS
ACTUALLY DRY TO EAT.

ANCIENT, REVERED SUPERFOOD

From the Andean valleys of Peru comes a fruit known as the Gold of the Incas, revered by the ancient Incas for its delicious flavor and nutritional density.

Lucuma provides fourteen essential trace elements, including a considerable amount of potassium, sodium, calcium, magnesium, and phosphorus. The bright yellow fruit has a dry flesh, which possesses a unique flavor somewhat like maple, caramel custard, and sweet potato, with a smooth consistency that melts in your mouth.

HOW WE USE LUCUMA POWDER

Lucuma powder has a pleasantly sweet taste that can be described as rich, creamy, and malty. In its raw powder form, lucuma can be used as a natural and nutritious sweetener. It is an excellent flavoring for raw chocolates and smoothies.

THE MAGIC OF LUCUMA

NUTRIENT RICH

LOW-GI SWEETENER

IMMUNE ENHANCING

INCREASED ENERGY

Nutrient rich

Lucuma is an excellent source of carbohydrates, fiber, and vitamins, especially betacarotene, niacin, and vitamin C. It is also a good source of minerals such as calcium and phosphorus and has high concentrations of iron. It also has 92 mg of calcium per 100 g, to keep your bones and teeth strong. Phosphorus is important for bone and protein formation.

Low-GI sweetener

The combination of complex carbohydrates, minerals, and fiber make it an excellent low-GI addition to recipes.

Immune enhancing

The carotenoids in lucuma have powerful antioxidant and immune-enhancing properties that promote proper cell communication. The iron in lucuma may help stimulate the immune system and improve physical endurance.

Increased energy

As lucuma is a good source of iron, regular consumption can also increase energy levels in the body, thanks to proper oxygenation of the blood.

LUCUMA RECIPES

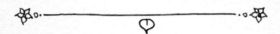

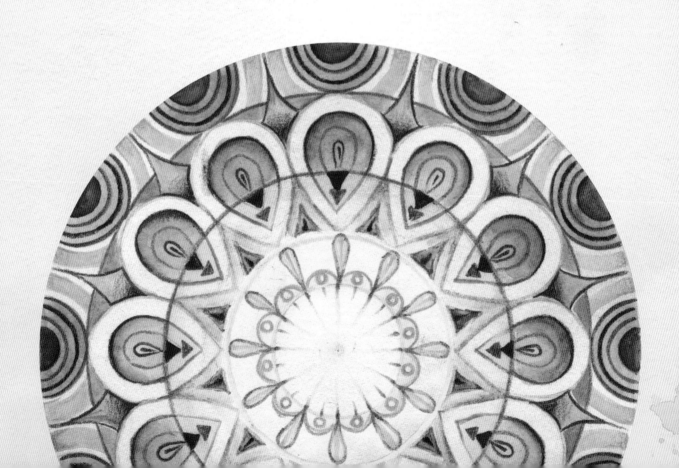

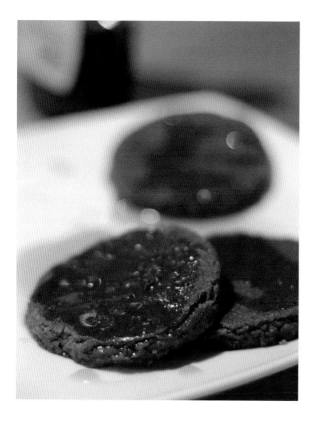

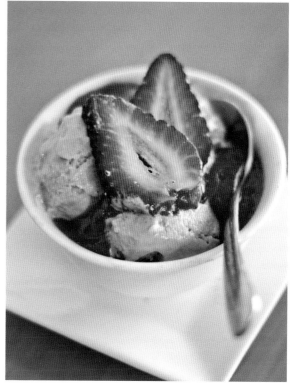

LUCUMA FLAPJACKS

Serves 2–4

¾ C oat flour (take rolled oats and grind fine into powder)

½ C lucuma powder

¼ C yacon powder

¼ C honey

¼ C cacao butter

2 T maca

1 t vanilla extract

¼ t salt

1½ C warm water

Powderize the oats in a food processor first. Then add the remaining ingredients and blend smooth. Spread out onto a dehydrator teflex sheet and dry for six hours. After the first two hours, flip off the solid sheet and dry for the remaining four hours. Cut into rounds and enjoy with honey and chia omega cream (see page 64).

LUCUMA ICE CREAM

Makes ½ qt

1 C water

1 banana

¼ C lucuma powder

¼ C white mulberries

2 T honey

½ C cashews

Blend all ingredients together in a high-speed blender and freeze.

TROPICAL FRUIT SMOOTHIE

Makes 1 qt

> 1 C water or coconut water
> 1 banana, frozen
> 1 mango or ½ pineapple
> 3 passion fruits
> ⅛ C lucuma powder
> juice of 1 orange

Blend and enjoy.

CREAMY LUCUMA AND PAPAYA BREAKFAST

Serves 2–4

> 1 papaya
> 2 C hemp milk (see page 131)
> ¼ C lucuma powder
> juice of 1 lemon
> a handful of gojis

Blend the papaya with the hemp milk, lucuma powder, and lemon juice. Serve with a handful of gojis on top.

LUCUMA CUSTARD

Serves 2–4

> 1 C warm water
> ½ C cashews
> 2 bananas
> ¾ C lucuma powder
> 1 T honey
> ½ t vanilla extract
> a pinch of salt
> 1 mango (when in season)

Blend in a power blender and serve.

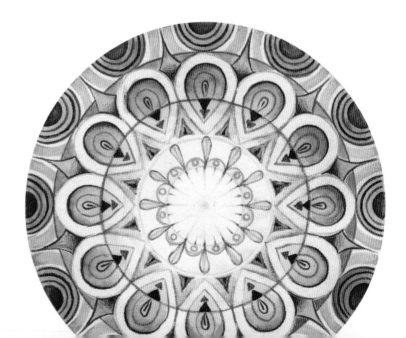

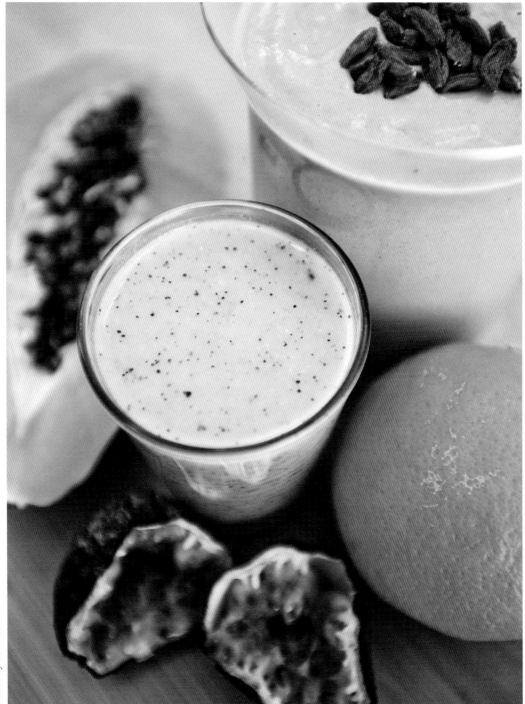

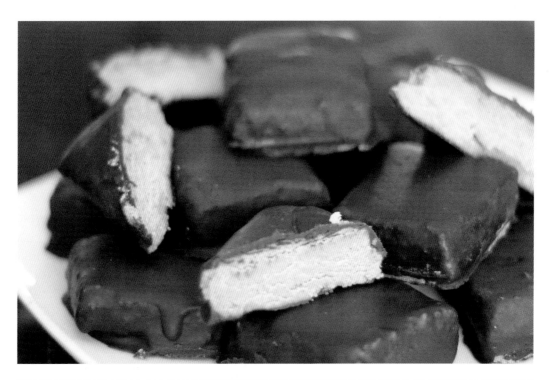

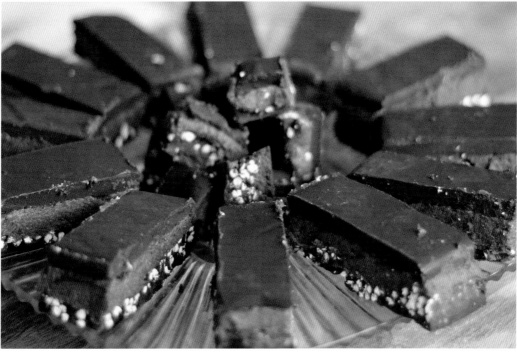

LUCUMA FUDGE

Melt cacao butter and then blend all ingredients in a high-speed blender until smooth. If it looks curdled, add a little more water. Shape into a big flat square on a teflex sheet about half an inch high. Allow to set in the freezer until firm for about 1 hour.

Remove and cut into squares. Dip in raw chocolate sauce and set in the fridge.

Makes 20–25 squares

>*2 C cacao butter, melted*
>*1 C lucuma powder*
>*½ C honey*
>*a pinch of salt*
>*¾ C water*
>*chocolate sauce for dipping*
>*(see page 229)*

JOSHUA'S BAR NONES

Josh, who is now ten years old and loves making chocolates with me, came over a short while ago and wanted to make "Bar Nones." We put our heads together and had a blast making these chocolates with a lucuma caramel filling and vanilla buckwheat crunch. We ate so much chocolate that day!

These Bar Nones can be made without the vanilla buckwheaties, but they add a lovely extra crunch. You will have to make the buckwheaties the day before, or make a double batch and store them in a glass jar in your kitchen. You can use the buckwheaties in a variety of chocolate recipes or as an addition to breakfast cereals with nut milk.

For the vanilla buckwheaties, combine the buckwheat with the honey and vanilla. Dehydrate for 12 hours or until crispy.

Line a rectangular baking tin with parchment paper.

Pour in one portion of chocolate sauce as the base layer. Allow to set in the fridge while you make up the lucuma caramel.

Blend the dates, lucuma powder, vanilla powder, and honey together in a high-speed blender until a nice stiff paste is formed. You can add a little water if the mixture is too hard to work the ingredients through nicely.

Spread caramel over the chocolate layer. Add a layer of vanilla buckwheaties. Pour the second portion of the chocolate sauce over the top and allow to set in the fridge. Once set, remove the parchment paper and slice into long bars or squares.

This is exceptionally rich and decadent!

Makes 20–25 bars

For the vanilla buckwheaties:

>*2 C buckwheat, soaked for 20 minutes and rinsed*
>*¼ C honey*
>*1 T vanilla extract*

For the chocolate:

>*2 portions of chocolate sauce recipe (see page 229)*

For the lucuma caramel filling:

>*1 C dates, soaked*
>*¾ C lucuma powder*
>*1 t vanilla powder*
>*¼ C honey*

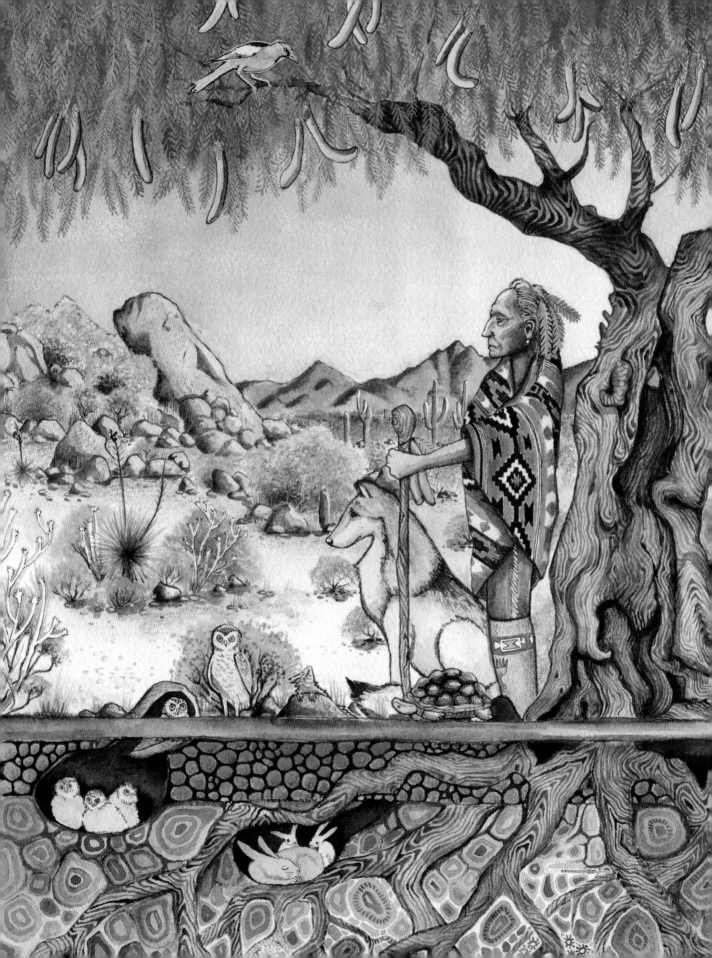

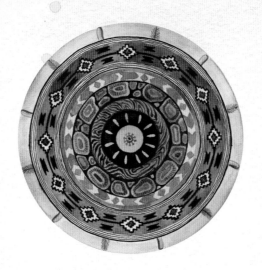

MESQUITE

NATIVE AMERICAN WHITE CAROB

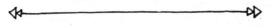

BLOOD SUGAR BALANCING

PROTEIN RICH

ANTI-ANXIETY

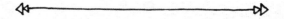

Shade in the desert, a versatile bean,
Giving flour, drink, and syrup for people to glean,
Standing and witnessing, Spirit of Mesquite,
Wooden staff in his hand and soft boots on his feet,
Animal companions, and all things that grow,
Roots that reach down and do wonders below:
A soil community that they support and nourish
Fixing nitrogen in the soil so that more life can flourish.
Elder of Mesquite, who cares for the clay,
If we follow your footsteps, and copy your way,
With our eyes and our hearts we will see in the loam
Our substance reflected, and a place we call home.

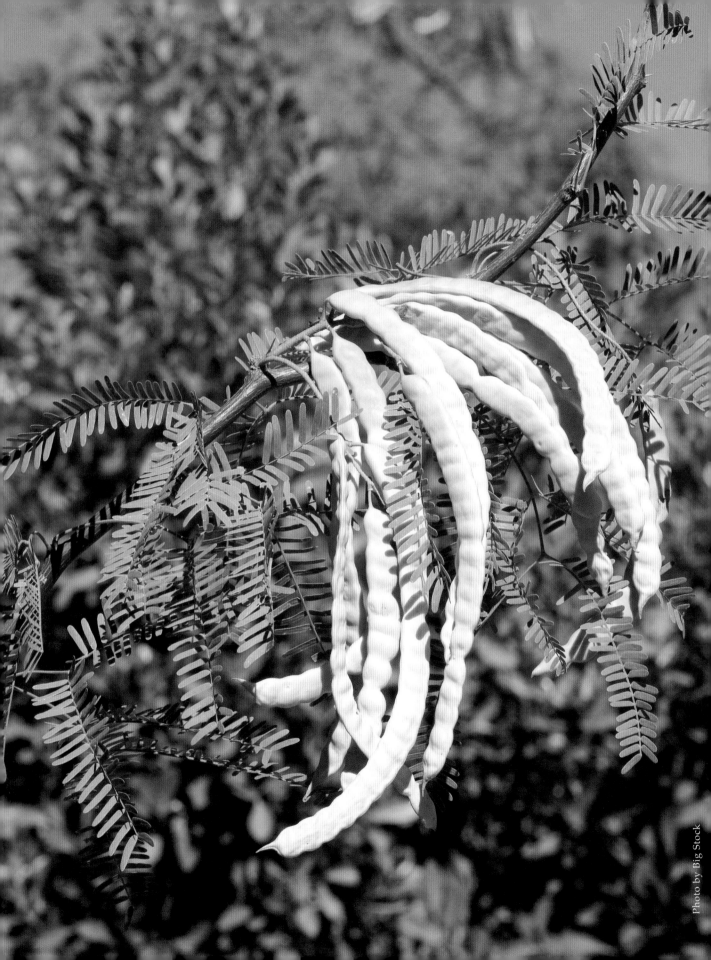

ANCIENT, REVERED SUPERFOOD

Mesquite pods are among the earliest known foods of prehistoric humans in the New World. Native Americans saw it as an integral part of their culture. The tree was relied on for a myriad of necessities such as food, weapons, shelter, and medicine, and they drew upon mesquite in almost every aspect of their lives. The bean pods served as food and were used to make medicinal tea.

The mesquite tree is a relative of carob, and mesquite is often called Peruvian carob. The tree is a nitrogen fixer, nitrifying dry arid regions to support more life. It's one of the few trees that thrives in the desert heat. It has no known insect or disease pests and spreads readily by seeds or sprouting from its crown. The seed pods are ground into flour, and are rich in protein. They contain L-lysine as well as calcium, magnesium, potassium, iron, and zinc.

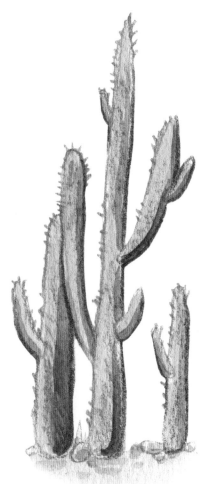

THE MAGIC OF MESQUITE

BLOOD SUGAR BALANCING

PROTEIN RICH

ANTI-ANXIETY

Blood sugar balancing

Mesquite is highly effective in balancing blood sugar. The natural sweetness in the pods comes from fructose, which doesn't require insulin in order to be metabolized, making it safe for diabetics. It also has a low GI of 25. Rich in galactomannans (soluble fibers), the nutrients in mesquite are absorbed slowly, effectively balancing blood sugar and preventing hunger.

Protein rich

At 17% protein, mesquite is an excellent protein source. Its protein content is higher than nearly every grain and many nuts and seeds.

Anti-anxiety

The presence of L-lysine supports the reduction of anxiety, and the rich tryptophan content supports the brain's stress-defense shield.

HOW WE USE MESQUITE POWDER

Mesquite has a sweet, slightly nutty flavor, with a hint of molasses. It can be used as a natural and nutritious sweetener in recipes and is an excellent flavoring for smoothies, snack bars, granola, raw chocolates, and desserts.

MESQUITE RECIPES

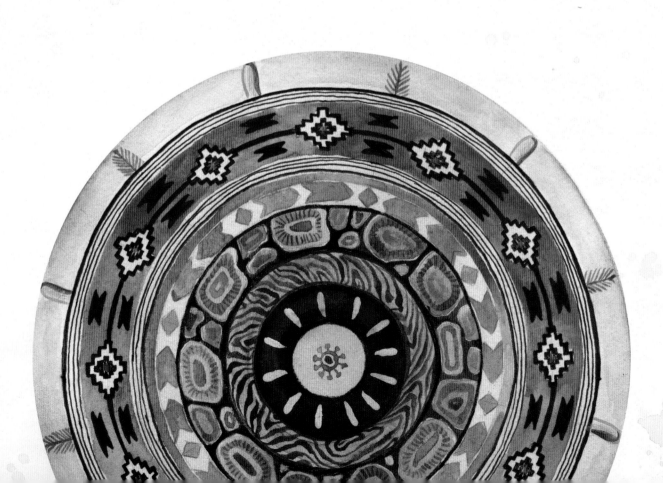

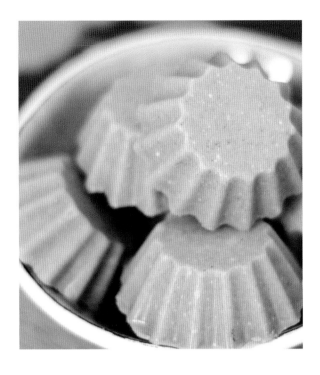

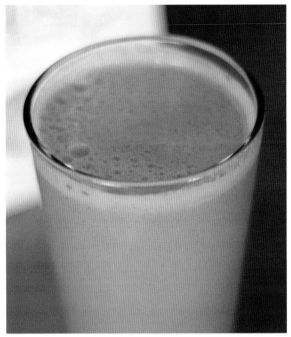

MESQUITE AND LUCUMA WHITE CHOCOLATES

  1 C cashews
  1 C cacao butter, melted
  ¼ C coconut oil, melted
  ¼ C honey
  2 T mesquite
  1 T lucuma powder
  ½ t vanilla extract

Place cashews in a high-speed blender and quickly blend to powderize them. Add the melted cacao butter and coconut oil and blend until smooth. On slow speed, add the honey, mesquite, lucuma powder, and vanilla extract. Pour into molds and set in the fridge.

Beware: Overblending chocolates on high speed can "shock" your chocolates and make the oils separate from the solids. If you do this by mistake, pop your mixture into the fridge as it makes delicious toffee.

Tip: Adding vanilla buckwheaties would raise the bar on these already delicious chocolates (see page 189).

MEDICINAL MESQUITE AND CHOCOLATE SMOOTHIE

Experiment with supercharging your smoothies with superherbs.

Makes 1 qt

  3 C water
  ¼ C Brazil nuts
  ¼ C white mulberries
  ¼ C cacao powder
  3 T honey
  2 T mesquite powder
  2 T chia seeds
  1 T maca powder
  1 t ashwagandha
  1 t foti

Blend all ingredients together.

PERUVIAN OAT BARS

Makes 25 bars

    2 C dates
    2 C warm water
    ½ C cacao powder
    3 C oats
    1 C mesquite
    1 C lucuma powder
    1 C raisins
    ½ C cacao nibs
    ½ C chia, ground
    ¼ C maca
    1 T vanilla powder
    ½ t salt
    chocolate sauce for dipping
       (see page 229)

This power bar combines the strength of many of the Peruvian superfoods. They are great to have with you on hikes.

Soak the dates in the water for 15 minutes.

Blend the dates and the soak water into a date jam, adding the cacao powder to make it a chocolate date jam.

In a food processor, pulse the oats until roughly chopped and then add all remaining ingredients except for the chocolate sauce and pulse. Place dry ingredients in a bowl and add the date jam. Work it through into a doughy consistency. Spread out onto a teflex sheet and dry in a dehydrator for 12 hours. Cut into bar shapes and dip into chocolate sauce. Allow the chocolate to set in the fridge.

SUPER-GRANOLA

Fills a 3-qt jar

For the paste:

    3 C warm water
    2 C dates, pitted
    2 C cashews or Brazil nuts
    ½ C mesquite powder
    1 T vanilla powder
    1 t cinnamon
    1 t salt

For the mixture:

    4 C mixed seeds and nuts
    4 C rolled oats or buckwheat,
       activated and dried

This recipe comes from Natalie Reid and Noel Marten's raw recipe book *Easy Living Food,* and it is loaded with superfoods. The mesquite adds sweetness as well as a delicious, creamy, malty flavor. Natalie made an enormous batch of this granola when we went on our road trip around the country with David Wolfe. It is delicious with nut milk and fruit. It was a tour hit!

Soak the dates in the water for 15 minutes.

Blend the dates and all the paste ingredients until smooth.

For the mixture, roughly break up the seeds and nuts—either in the processor or put them in a tough bag and tap with a chopping board until broken up.

Add everything into a bowl and stir well until all is well coated. Dry for 12 hours on solid sheets, then dry on mesh trays for a further 36 hours until completely crisp.

BANANA BREAD

Serves 4–6

    1 C almonds, soaked
    ½ C mesquite
    2 bananas
    ¼ C chia seeds
    ¼ C yacon powder
    ½ C desiccated coconut
    ½ t vanilla powder
    ½ C water

This banana bread is lovely served with nut butter and honey.

Grind the almonds in a food processor. Then add the remaining ingredients to the food processor, reserving the water until last and adding it slowly until a doughy ball is formed. Shape into a loaf and place in the dehydrator. Dry for 8–12 hours.

Slice and serve with honey.

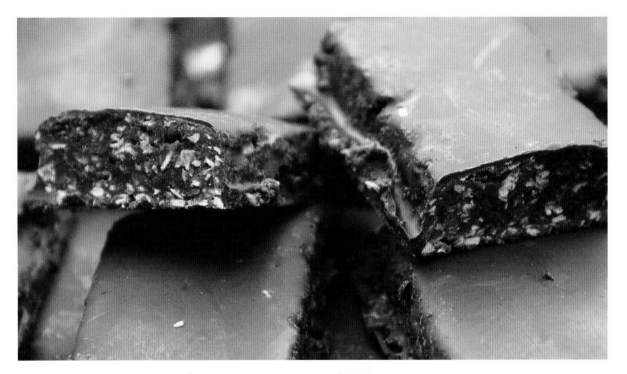

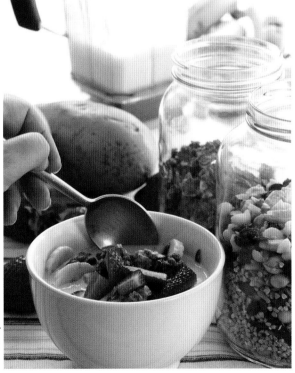

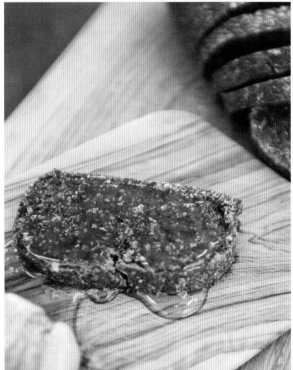

Photo by Luke Daniel

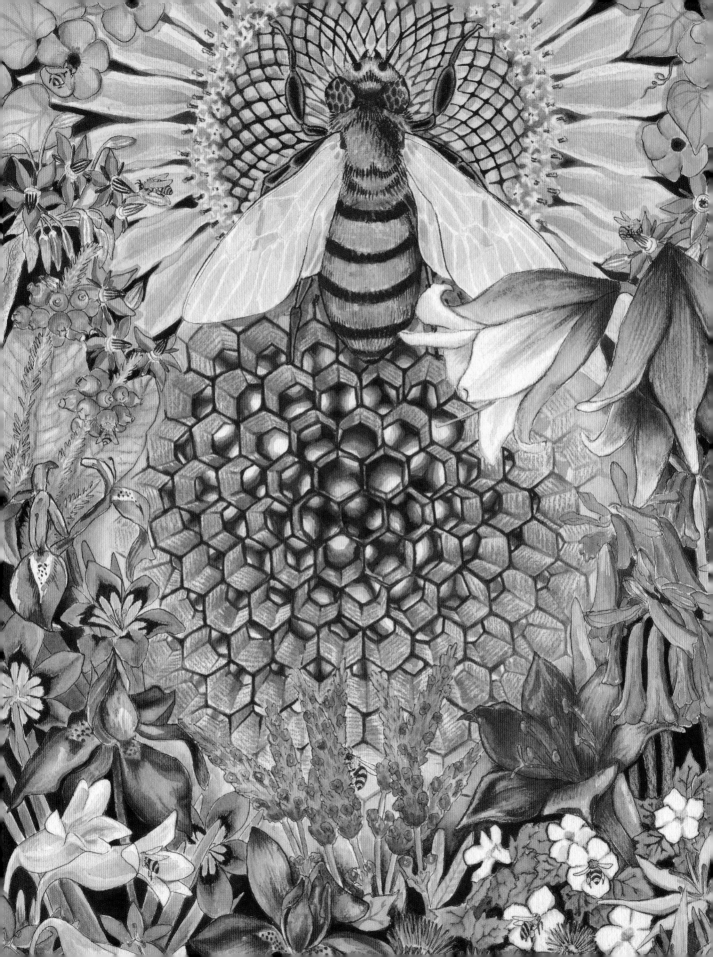

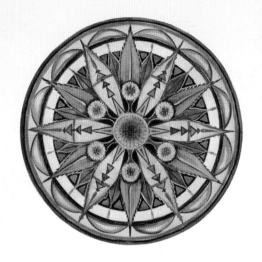

BEE PRODUCTS

DISTILLED SUNSHINE

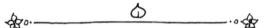

ENERGY ENHANCER • SKIN HEALER • TREATING ALLERGIES • DIGESTIVE HEALTH

IMMUNE SYSTEM BOOSTER • CARDIOVASCULAR HEALTH • ANTIVIRAL

ANTI-TUMOR • BLOOD SUGAR BALANCING • LONGEVITY

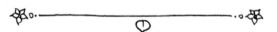

An ocean of color, faces turned to the sun,
Flowers open their petals, the day has begun.
Next, on the air, there's a humming of wings,
A ritual that is a most ancient of things . . .
Working together, a hive that's one mind,
Harvesting from all of the blooms that they find,
Bees fetch nectar and pollen, which they carry back home
Where they process their bounty 'round the honeycomb . . .
Geometric matrix, hexagonally crafted
By a humming intelligence as carefully drafted,
Propolis, royal jelly, pollen, and wax
All made on the bees' small, industrious backs.
And of course golden honey like sunlight suspended
A magical syrup—decomposition transcended.
From sunlight to flowers to bees to mankind
We may share in the magic that they have refined.

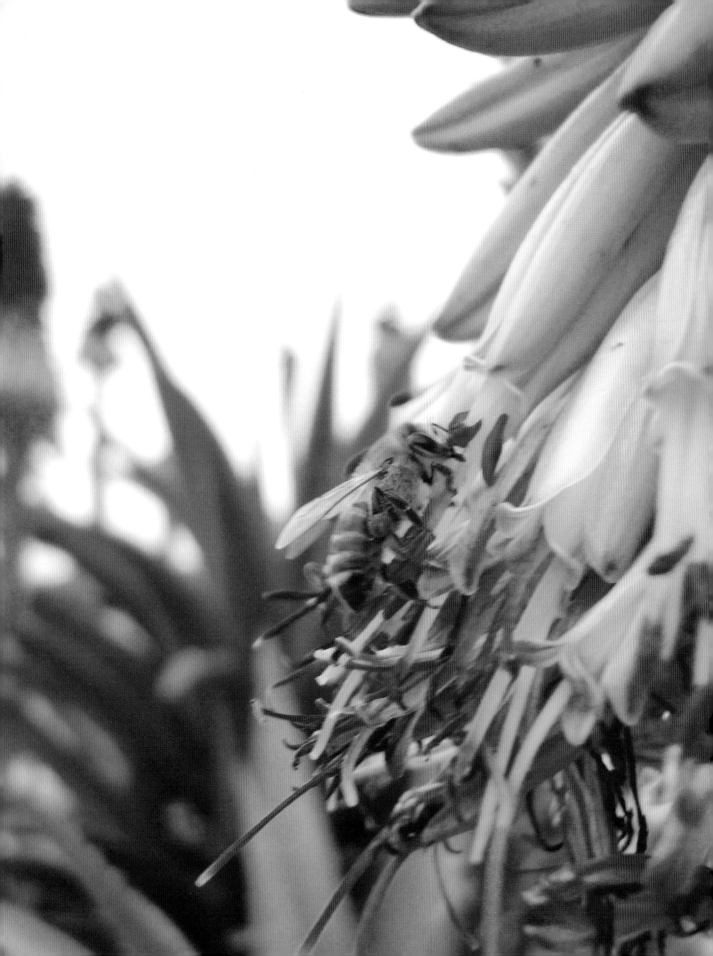

ANCIENT, REVERED SUPERFOOD

History, legend, and mythology surrounding bees and bee products stretch back into the prehistoric era. From ancient Egypt to ancient Greece, bee products have been revered for their healing and nutritional benefits. Honeybees are the only insects that produce food that is synergistic with humans. They are magical, mysterious creatures capable of incredible feats. A hive of bees will fly 93,205 miles, the equivalent of three orbits around the earth, to collect 2.2 lb of honey! A worker bee lives for only three to six weeks and visits up to a thousand flowers a day. The brain of a worker honeybee is about a cubic millimeter, yet has the densest neurological tissue of any animal. Bees produce the only food that will never spoil. Edible honey has even been found in Egyptian tombs.

Bee products are available as raw honey, bee pollen, royal jelly, and propolis.

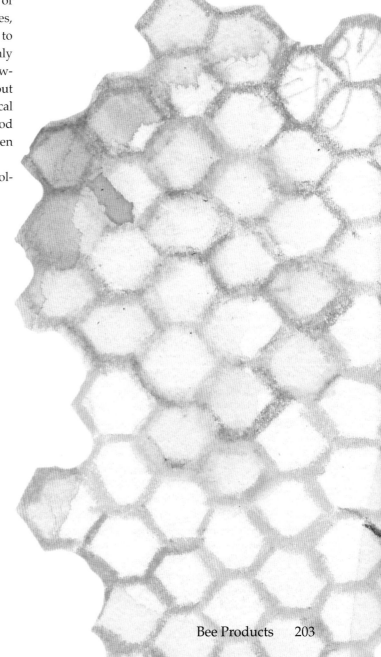

THE ONLY INSECT THAT PRODUCES SOMETHING THAT A HUMAN CAN EAT IS THE HONEYBEE.

Raw honey

Raw honey is honey in its purest, natural form. Honey collection is an ancient activity. Humans apparently began hunting for honey at least 8,000 years ago, as evidenced by a cave painting in Valencia, Spain. Raw honey is nature's own multivitamin. Raw honey is a natural source of vitamins B1, B2, B3, B5, and B6, and even antioxidant-rich vitamin C. It also contains minerals such as magnesium, potassium, calcium, sodium chloride, sulfur, and phosphate.

Bees feast on flowers, collecting the flower nectar in their mouths. This nectar then mixes with special enzymes in the bees' saliva, a process that turns it into honey. Bees carry the honey back to the hive, where they deposit it into the cells of the hive's walls. The fluttering of their wings provides the necessary ventilation to reduce the moisture content, making it ready for consumption.

The health benefits of consuming honey appear in Greek, Roman, Vedic, and Islamic texts. The healing qualities of honey were referred to by philosophers and scientists all the way back to ancient times, such as Aristotle (384–322 BCE) and Aristoxenus (320 BCE).

Bee pollen

Bee pollen is considered to be the most complete food found in nature. Pollen is the male seed of a flower blossom, which is collected by honeybees and mixed with the bees' digestive enzymes. Bee pollen is a blend of sticky pollen granules that contain up to five million pollen spores each. Revered by many scientists as a complete, nutritionally perfect food, these tiny pollens contain almost all the nutrients required by the human body. They are enormously rich in proteins, vitamins, minerals, beneficial fatty acids, carotenoids, and bioflavonoids. They are antiviral, antibacterial, and helpful in lowering cholesterol as well as stabilizing and strengthening capillaries.

Royal jelly

Royal jelly is a creamy white or pale yellowish substance specially created by worker bees. They mix honey and bee pollen with enzymes in the glands of their throats to produce this extraordinary food. All bee larvae are fed royal jelly mouth to mouth by the worker bees, for the first three or four days after hatching. The queen eats nothing but this perfect food throughout her adult life, and can live eight to ten times as long as the simple worker bee, which typically has a lifespan of only about three to six weeks. Royal jelly contains an extraordinarily high concentration of vitamins B5 and B6, and amino acids, and is believed to be a potent antioxidant and a special rejuvenating substance that promotes tissue growth and muscle and cell regeneration.

Propolis

Certain trees produce sticky resins as part of their immune system to defend themselves against disease. Bees collect the resin that oozes from the buds of plants. The bees chew these substances and mix them with their saliva and other substances to form propolis. It is created to sterilize the hive and protect it against diseases and infection. In fact, "propolis" means "in defense of the city" in Greek. Not only does it help inhibit the spread of bacteria, viruses, and fungi in the hive, it also helps fight against climatic changes. It is used as a "putty" to seal cracks and openings in the hive and to strengthen and repair honeycombs, and for this reason is also known as "bee glue." It is especially rich in amino acids, has a high vitamin content including vitamins A, B1, B2, and B3, and biotin, and is extremely rich in bioflavonoids, which are believed to have numerous immune-building properties and health benefits. It provides protection against infectious invaders and promotes healing and regeneration of tissue. It is used in ointments for healing cuts and wounds and has been shown to have outstanding value for treating a wide variety of illnesses. It is also used as a natural alternative to penicillin and other antibiotics.

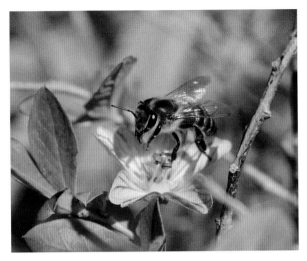

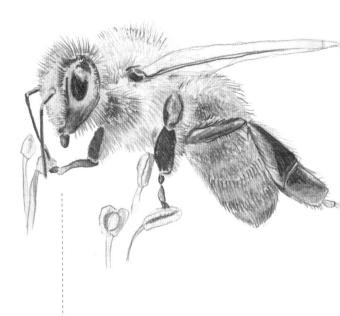

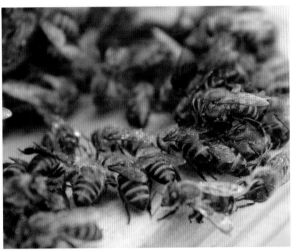

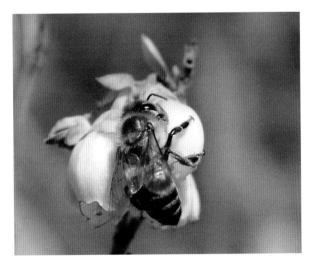

DURING ITS LIFETIME, AN AVERAGE HONEYBEE PRODUCES ONE-TWELFTH OF A TEASPOON OF HONEY.

EIGHTY PERCENT OF POLLINATION WITHIN NATURE IS DONE BY THE HONEYBEE.

A HONEYBEE VISITS 50 TO 100 FLOWERS DURING A COLLECTION TRIP.

THE MAGIC OF BEE PRODUCTS

- ENERGY ENHANCER
- SKIN HEALER
- TREATING ALLERGIES
- DIGESTIVE HEALTH
- IMMUNE SYSTEM BOOSTER
- CARDIOVASCULAR HEALTH
- ANTIVIRAL
- ANTI-TUMOR
- BLOOD SUGAR BALANCING
- LONGEVITY

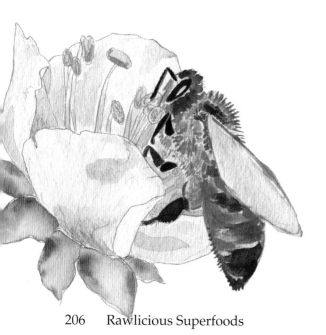

Energy enhancer

The range of nutrients found within bee products makes them a great natural energizer. The carbohydrates, protein, and B vitamins can help keep you going all day by enhancing stamina and fighting off fatigue. Honey is the ideal liver fuel because it contains a nearly 1:1 ratio of fructose to glucose. Fructose "unlocks" an enzyme from the liver cell's nucleus that is necessary for the incorporation of glucose into glycogen (the form in which sugar is stored in the liver and muscle cells). An adequate glycogen store in the liver is essential to supply the brain with fuel during sleeping and prolonged exercise.

Skin healer

Honey has been used topically as an antiseptic therapeutic agent for the treatment of ulcers, burns, and wounds for centuries. Honey is a good skin moisturizer and effectively tones and firms up the skin. Bee pollen is often used in topical products that aim to treat inflammatory conditions and common skin irritations such as psoriasis or eczema. The amino acids and vitamins protect the skin and aid the regeneration of cells.

Treating allergies

Pollen reduces the presence of histamine, improving many allergies. Dr. Leo Conway, MD, of Denver, Colorado, reported that 94% of his patients were completely free from allergy symptoms once treated with oral feeding of pollen. Everything from asthma to allergies to sinus problems was cleared, confirming that bee pollen is wonderfully effective against a wide range of respiratory diseases.

Digestive health

In addition to healthful vitamins, minerals, and protein, bee pollen and honey contain enzymes that aid digestion. Enzymes assist your body to get all the nutrients you need from the food that you eat. There are more than 100 active enzymes present in fresh and unheated pollens and honey. Eating foods that contain enzymes helps the body prevent and fight diseases such as cancer and arthritis, and saves the body from having to make enzymes, a process that depletes energy. Different varieties of honey also possess a large amount of friendly bacteria (six species of lactobacilli and four species of bifidobacteria), which support digestive health. Recent research shows that honey treatment may help disorders such as ulcers and bacterial gastroenteritis.

Immune system booster

Pollen is good for the intestinal flora and thereby supports the immune system. Bee products have antibiotic-type properties that can help protect the body from viruses. They are also rich in antioxidants that protect the cells from the damaging oxidation of free radicals.

Cardiovascular health

Bee pollen contains large amounts of rutin, an antioxidant bioflavonoid that helps strengthen capillaries and blood vessels, assists with circulatory problems, and corrects cholesterol levels. Its potent anti-clotting powers could help prevent heart attacks and strokes.

Antiviral

All honey is antibacterial, antiviral, and antifungal because the bees add an enzyme that makes hydrogen peroxide. One of the best-known health benefits of honey is its ability to soothe sore throats and kill the bacteria that causes the infection.

Anti-tumor

Other phytonutrients found both in honey and propolis have been shown to possess cancer-preventing and anti-tumor properties. These substances include caffeic acid, methyl caffeate, phenylethyl caffeate, and phenylethyl dimethylcaffeate. Researchers have discovered that these substances prevent colon cancer in animals by shutting down the activity of two enzymes, phosphatidylinositol-specific phospholipase C and lipoxygenase.

Blood sugar balancing

Evidence indicates that consumption of raw honey may improve blood sugar control and insulin sensitivity compared to other sweeteners. The body's tolerance to raw honey is significantly better than to sucrose or glucose alone. Despite containing more calories than sugar (twenty-one per teaspoon versus sixteen), it's unlikely to expand your waistline: A recent study found that overweight or obese patients who received a 2.5-ounce dose of honey every day for a month lowered both their total and LDL cholesterol, while they maintained or even lost weight.

Longevity

Centenarians have been found to consistently eat honey. The abundance of nutrients in bee products is deeply rejuvenating to the whole body and promotes cellular longevity. The high antioxidant levels in bee pollen help increase longevity by neutralizing free radicals.

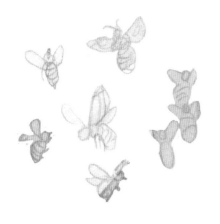

QUALITY IS KEY

Honey and high heat do not get along very well. It has been found that excessive heat can have detrimental effects on the nutritional value of honey. Heating up honey to 98.6°F (37°C) causes loss of nearly 200 components, some of which are antibacterial. Heating up to 104°F (40°C) destroys invertase, an important enzyme. At 122°F (50°C), the honey sugars caramelize, and it turns from a light color to an increasingly darker color as the temperature rises. When honey is excessively heated, micron-filtered, and/or pasteurized (usually at 170.6°F/77°C), nearly all the beneficial components of honey are removed.

HOW WE USE BEE PRODUCTS

Raw honey

As beekeepers ourselves, we are conscious of minimizing the stress experienced by the bees while harvesting some of their precious food. Commercial beekeepers will often over-harvest honey and keep the bees alive on sugar water during winter when they have no food. Only buy bee products from beekeepers who are conscious and considerate in how they treat their bees. Go to farmers' markets and chat with the beekeeper directly to be sure. The quality of honey is a function of the plants and environment from which pollen, saps, nectars, and resins were gathered. Other substances found in the environment—including traces of heavy metals, pesticides, and antibiotics—have been shown to appear in honey. The amount varies greatly. This is why we prefer *wild raw* honeys, usually harvested from hives located away from intensive farming.

We use raw honey in drinks, smoothies, drizzled over breakfast, in dressings, desserts, and, of course, in chocolate! We collect bottles of honey like some people collect bottles of wine. We love dipping straight into the different bottles we collect both from our own hives and from different areas—each unique honey offering different qualities and properties based on the flowers that grew in that area. Honeycomb is a special treat, with the added bonus of a waxy, natural chewing gum.

MOST HONEY AVAILABLE IN SUPERMARKETS IS PASTEURIZED AT HIGH TEMPERATURES. LOOK FOR HONEY THAT STATES THAT IT IS RAW. IF IN DOUBT, ASK IF IT HAS BEEN PASTEURIZED.

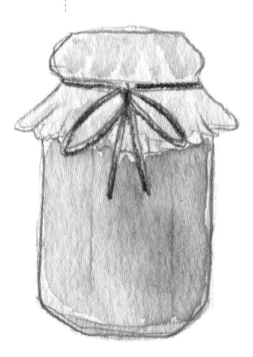

Bee pollen

High-quality fresh pollen consists of soft, fragrant, pliable granules that are neither pasteurized nor heated. These tiny yellow, orange, or brown granules dissolve on the tongue like magic. The taste of pollen varies depending on the flower and nectar source it comes from. Some pollen has a slightly sweet and nutty flavor, while some pollen tastes bitter. We eat bee pollen plain as an energy-boosting snack. As it is a very rich food, it is recommended that those who are new to it take a small dosage (about a quarter teaspoon) to start with. Then work up to one tablespoon of bee pollen each day for children or adults and thereafter increase the servings as desired. It is one of Katara's favorite first foods! It blends well with smoothies too. Don't cook with the granules or add powdered granules to anything that requires heat. Heat destroys the live enzymes and reduces the nutrient value. Conscious and considerate beekeepers are able to remove a small portion of the pollen from hives while leaving most for the bees and without harming the bees or disturbing their routine.

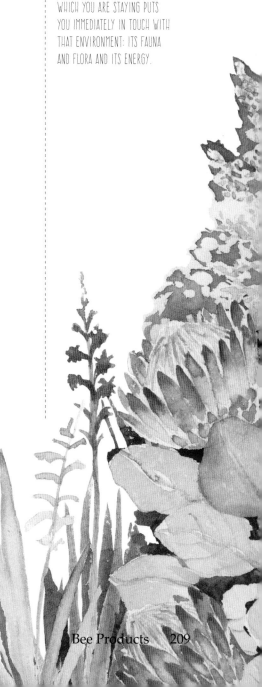

EATING HONEY FROM AN AREA IN WHICH YOU ARE STAYING PUTS YOU IMMEDIATELY IN TOUCH WITH THAT ENVIRONMENT: ITS FAUNA AND FLORA AND ITS ENERGY.

Royal jelly

Royal jelly is extremely potent. Use as little as half a teaspoon a day, mixed into food or eaten straight off the spoon.

Propolis

Propolis is usually sold in tincture form. It is an excellent skin healer and can also be used internally for infections.

WARNINGS

Do not feed honey-containing products or use honey as a flavoring for infants under one year of age. Honey may contain *Clostridium botulinum* spores and toxins that can cause infant botulism, a life-threatening paralytic disease. Honey is safe for children older than twelve months and adults.

Bee pollen is not the same as allergy-causing pollen that is dry, lightweight, and easily carried by the wind. Bee pollen will rarely cause allergy symptoms. However, people who are very cautious of allergic reactions could start with small amounts of pollen intake and gradually increase the amount.

BEE PRODUCT RECIPES

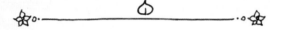

NUT BUTTER, HONEY, AND NIBS * ALMOND MILK AND HONEY
RAW HONEY * HONEYCOMB * BEE POLLEN

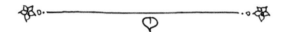

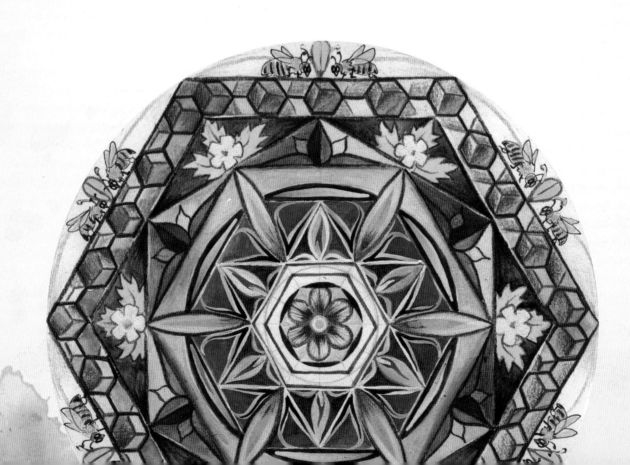

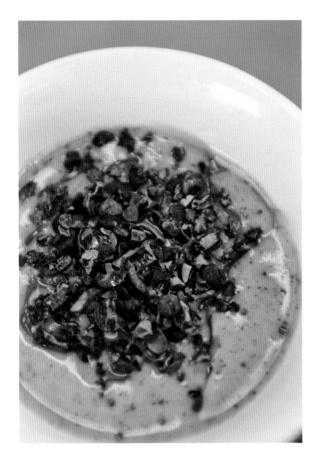

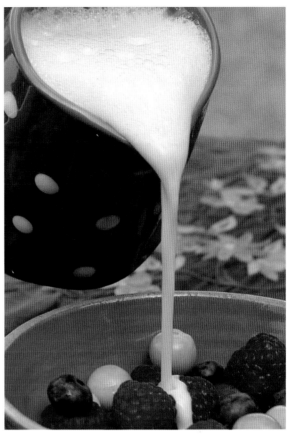

NUT BUTTER, HONEY, AND NIBS

Favorite 2-minute dessert.

> *raw nut butter of your choice*
> *raw honey of your choice (creamed honey is divine here)*
> *raw cacao nibs*

In a small bowl, combine all the ingredients and indulge in this scrumptious creamy dessert. It's even more decadent served with a bowl of fresh figs!

ALMOND MILK AND HONEY

Nut milks are essential to a raw food and/or superfoodist kitchen. Vary this recipe by replacing almonds with other nuts or seeds and adjusting honey for sweetness.

Makes 5 C

> *1 qt water*
> *1 C almonds, soaked and rinsed*
> *2 T honey*
> *1 vanilla pod or ¼ t vanilla extract*

Blend all the ingredients in a power blender and strain through a nut milk bag. Straining makes the liquid thinner and more "milk-like." You can leave this step out if you don't mind the extra creaminess of the nut pulp in your drink.

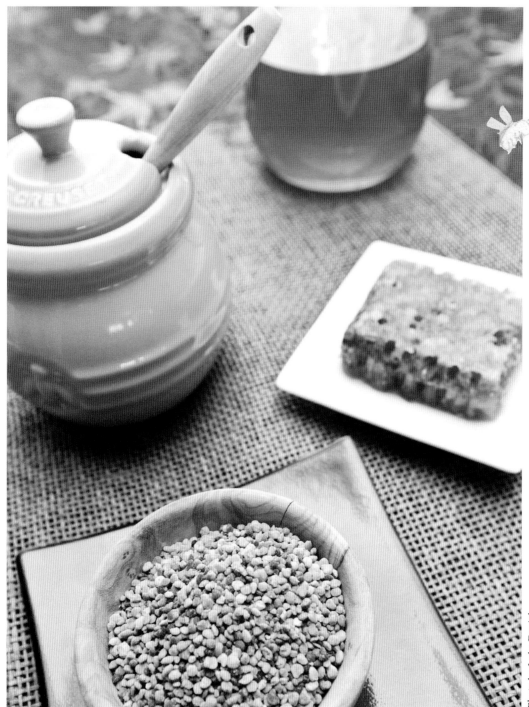

RAW HONEY

Raw honey is our sweetener of choice 90% of the time. You will find it scattered in many of the recipes throughout this book.

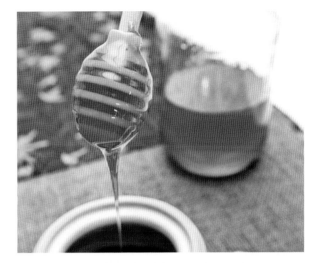

HONEYCOMB

The purest honey is from honeycomb, perfectly packed for freshness with the wax acting as a natural chewing gum.

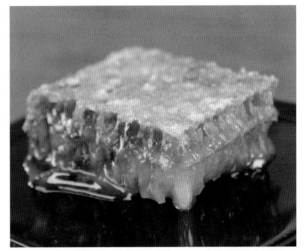

BEE POLLEN

You can eat bee pollen straight off the spoon—it's sweet and delicious. It's also lovely sprinkled on smoothies or over a fruit or chia breakfast.

Photos by Luke Daniel

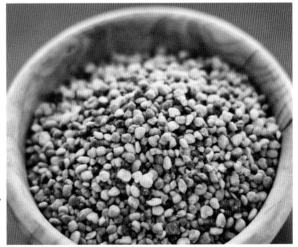

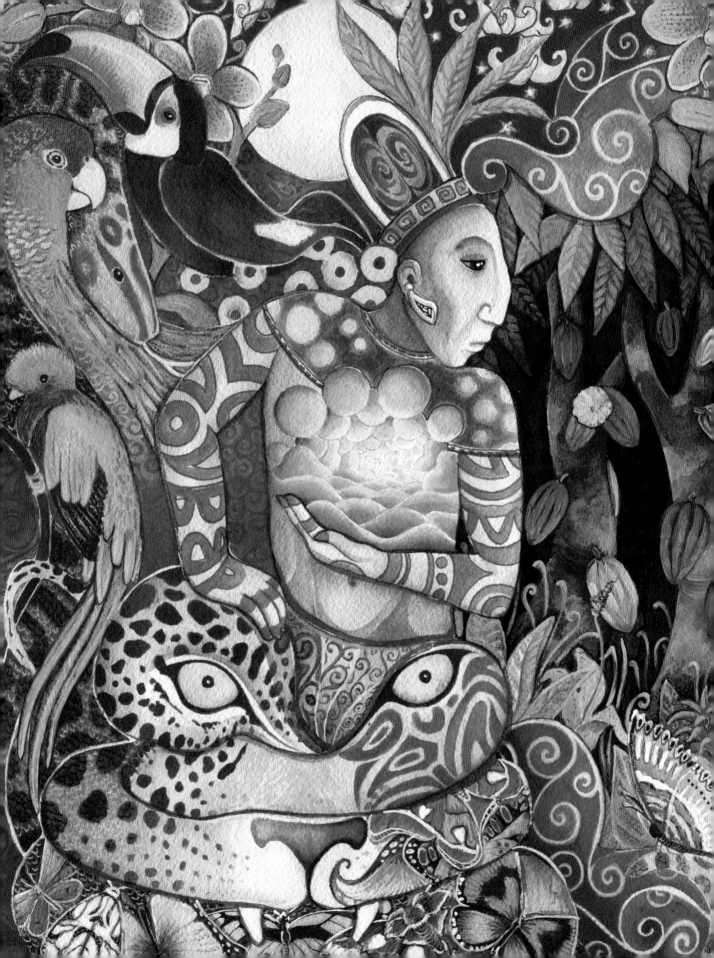

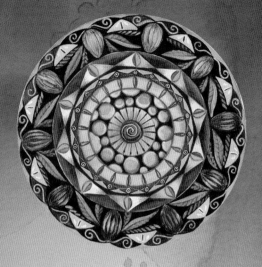

RAW CACAO

RAW CHOCOLATE: FOOD OF THE GODS

CARDIOVASCULAR HEALTH ∗ LONGEVITY ANTIOXIDANTS

BRAIN HEALTH ∗ ENERGY BOOSTING

NATURAL ANTIDEPRESSANT ∗ WEIGHT LOSS

Deep in a tree a human heart beats,
Deep in the jungle where everything meets,
A velvety presence, a midnight deep taste,
A lightening rhythm, with medicine laced.
Open your heart to the sound of the thrum
Of a celestial magic, an earthly hum,
An ascending dance through expanded mind,
A purple bean, beloved by mankind.
Cacao like a drumbeat, the pulse of elation
At work in your body to shift your vibration.
The Chocolate Shaman, the wielder of worlds,
Who sits where two realms meet, where mystery unfurls.

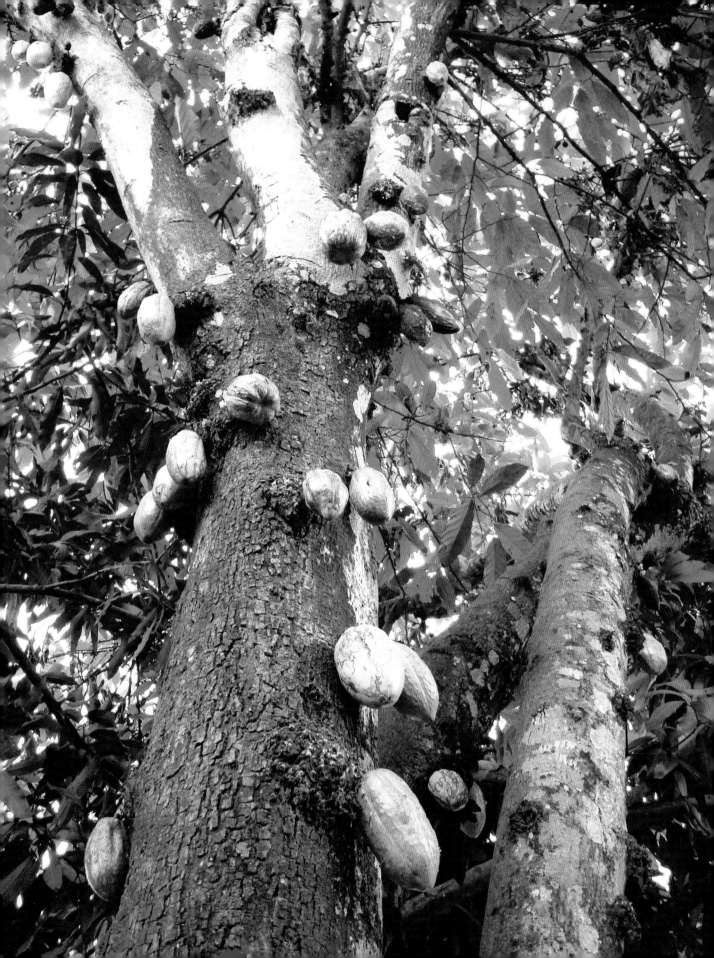

ANCIENT, REVERED SUPERFOOD

The cacao bean

Chocolate is one of the world's most loved foods, yet very few people have ever had the raw food that all chocolate comes from—cacao beans! Cacao beans are the seeds of the cacao fruit, which grows on a jungle tree. Botanically, cacao is actually a nut. The Latin name for this tree is *Theobroma cacao,* which literally translated means "cacao, the food of the gods." This is what the indigenous Central Americans used to call it.

THE CACAO TREE'S
BOTANICAL NAME IS
THEOBROMA CACAO,
WHICH MEANS "FOOD OF
THE GODS" IN GREEK.

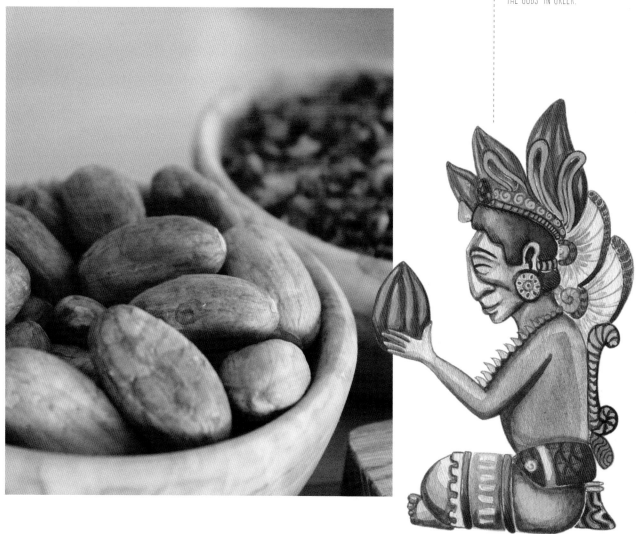

Money does grow on trees!

In ancient Central American cultures, raw cacao beans were used as money. Imagine: edible money! When the Spanish came, they called cacao "black gold" *(oro negro)* or "seeds of gold" *(pepas de oro)*. Cacao beans continued to be used as standard currency in Mexico until 1887. Cacao is wealth. Cacao embodies the energy of abundance and prosperity. This is the special, unique energy that makes cacao the most powerful food on earth.

A noble purple food

Cacao is a purple seed and, because of its high magnesium levels, it resonates with our heart and higher energy centers. It is associated with light-heartedness, fun, playfulness, and letting go. The Aztecs and Mayans associated it with nobility and abundance. The energy of cacao is wonderfully expressed in the original movie *Charlie and the Chocolate Factory*. Willie Wonka and his crew are fun, zany, and energetic, yet at the same time express a high level of integrity and wisdom. High-energy foods are easy to spot when using new technologies such as Kirlian photography. These foods show an incredibly high energetic vibration that far exceeds any standard food. Standard Western medicine and nutrition routinely overlook the importance of the energetic value and vibration of food.

Harvesting cacao

Unlike other fruits, cacao is always in season. The flowers are pollinated by midges and then develop into red, orange, green, purple, or yellow pods. The pods contain up to fifty cacao beans each, surrounded by sweet, white fruit flesh. The beans are harvested today in much the same way as they were by the Aztecs. After the pods ripen, which takes five to six months, they are removed from the tree and carefully cut open with a machete, and the cacao beans are extracted. After harvesting, the beans are placed

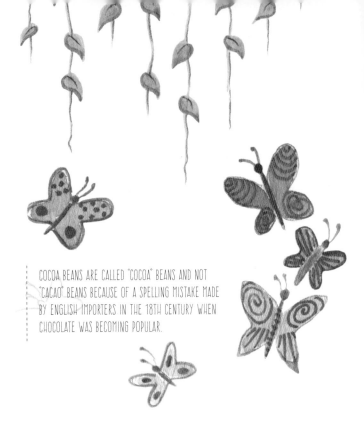

COCOA BEANS ARE CALLED "COCOA" BEANS AND NOT "CACAO" BEANS BECAUSE OF A SPELLING MISTAKE MADE BY ENGLISH IMPORTERS IN THE 18TH CENTURY WHEN CHOCOLATE WAS BECOMING POPULAR.

on banana leaves in large wooden boxes and left to ferment for a few days. During fermentation, the bitterness of the bean is reduced and the rich chocolate flavor begins to develop. The beans are then dried. During this drying process, the brown color develops and further flavor development occurs. Cacao contains an estimated 1,200 individual chemical constituents, making it one of the most complex food substances on earth! This complexity is why chocolate cannot be synthesized artificially.

Saving the planet with chocolate

The tropical rainforests of the planet are threatened by greed. The logging, mining, and oil industries are destroying our planet's most incredible resources. Since cacao enjoys the shade, it can be planted directly in the jungle without having to chop down all the trees. It can be a powerful buffer against deforestation. Unfortunately, with the increase in production of the CCN-51 hybrid, forests are no longer saved by all chocolate. Make sure you buy only heirloom varieties.

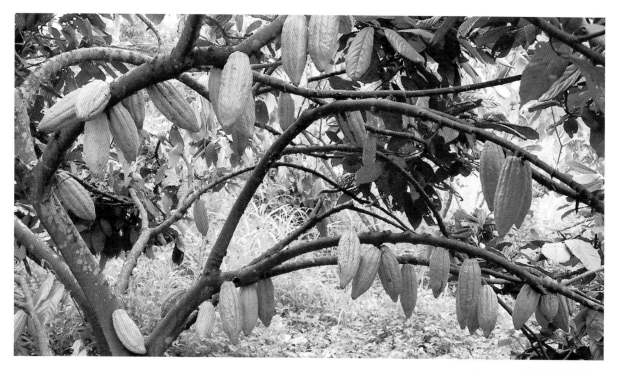

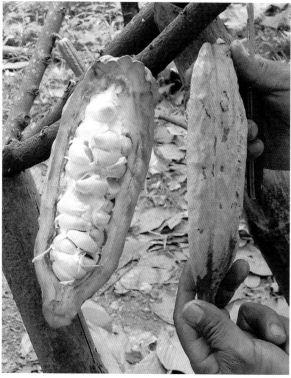

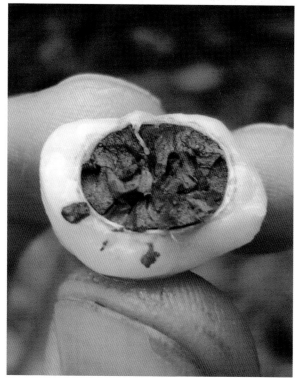

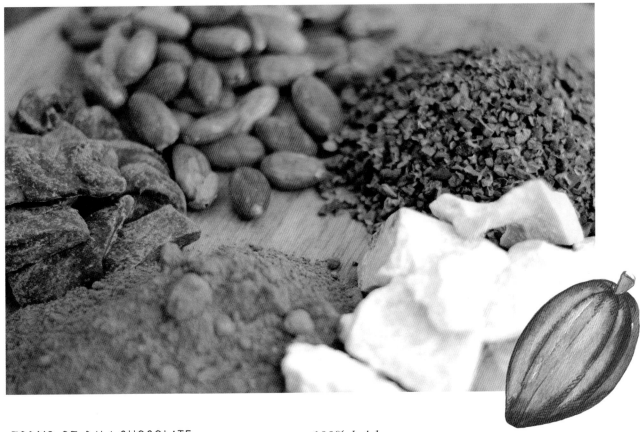

FORMS OF RAW CHOCOLATE

Cacao is available in five main forms that we can access and use in delicious raw food preparation.

Cacao beans are the original whole-food form of chocolate.

Cacao nibs are crushed cacao beans with the skins removed.

Chocolate liquor or paste is made by slowly grinding cacao nibs at low temperatures, resulting in warm, smooth, liquid cacao, which is then set.

Cacao butter is the fat of cold-pressed cacao nibs, and is solid at room temperature.

Cacao powder is the remaining cake after the butter has been pressed out. The cake is fine-milled.

100% heirloom raw cacao

Almost all commercially available chocolate has gone through a high-temperature roasting process that damages delicate vitamins, minerals, and antioxidants and causes the formation of trans fats and AGEs (advanced glycation end products). It's amazing that, even after all that, dark chocolate has still been shown to have certain health benefits, largely due to the nutritional density of the original food. Mass-produced chocolate, with dairy, sugar, and trans fats added, are in our view a toxic imposter of the original superfood.

Raw cacao is a superfood. The key to chocolate's super qualities seems to be found in eating it in its raw, natural state. Unfortunately most companies marketing raw chocolate don't do their homework on suppliers. They blindly accept stories about processing, and then unwittingly sell a product that

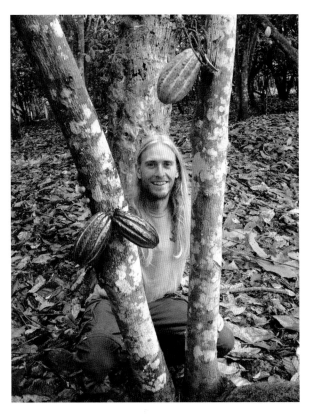
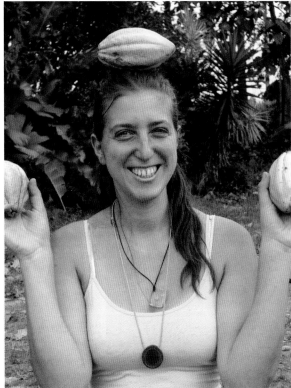

is labeled "raw" but that has actually been heated way above 113°F (45°C). Cacao powder and butter is usually never raw, as the friction of the machinery used to press the fat out can reach temperatures of over 212°F (100°C). There have also been cases of companies selling "raw" cacao that was loaded with molds, causing violent food poisoning and leading to many health enthusiasts claiming that raw cacao is not safe. We have had the opportunity to visit a truly raw cacao producer in Ecuador, seeing the growing, harvesting, and processing of the cacao done below 113°F (45°C) from start to end. It is much more expensive to process cacao at such low temperatures, as it takes much longer to make. This results in truly raw cacao products selling for higher prices than their cooked counterparts. At the end of the day, it is up to each person to decide if it is worth cutting corners for his or her wallet. We be-

lieve that the only option is to feed ourselves foods of the highest quality, integrity, and nutrient density.

There are three main strains of cacao used today in chocolate making. Forastero is the most grown, Criollo the least, and Trinitario is a hybrid between Criollo and Forastero. The heirloom Arriba Nacional bean of Ecuador is a regional Forastero variety that has a sweetness and unique fragrance different from other, often more bitter Forastero beans, and accounts for only 5% of the world's cacao harvested. This beautiful varietal, however, is being threatened by a hardy, aggressive, bland-flavored hybrid cacao called CCN-51, which is planted in full sun in rows like corn, destroying the natural forest that stood there before. It is widely used in the conventional chocolate industry.

HOW WE USE RAW CACAO

Cacao powder has a strong, rich, dark, bitter chocolate flavor. It's perfect for making raw chocolate desserts of all kinds. Blend into your favorite smoothies for a taste and health boost. Make your own healthy chocolates at home! The recommended daily intake is 5–20 g.

Cacao butter is the good fat or oil content of the cacao bean, which has been cold-pressed out of the bean. It allows one to make hard-set chocolates. You can also use it as an amazing skin moisturizer.

Cacao liquor or paste is made by slowly grinding down cacao nibs at low temperatures, resulting in warm, smooth, liquid cacao, which is then set. It allows you to make raw "snappy" chocolates that are solid at room temperature.

Cacao nibs have a strong, dark, bitter chocolate flavor. Sprinkle them over your morning breakfast or use them as chocolate chips in your smoothies. They can be ground into a rich dark powder using a coffee grinder to make raw desserts of all kinds. Add them to a trail or snack mix with goji berries and raisins. The recommended daily intake is 5–20 g or a small handful.

Cacao beans are the whole cacao bean. You can eat them whole—plain or dipped into raw honey. Blend them into your favorite smoothies or add them to snack mixes. The skins are edible, so you don't need to peel them first. The recommended daily intake is 5–20 whole beans.

Most people are used to eating chocolate sweet. Sweeteners, especially refined and processed sugars, are detrimental to our health and should be avoided. Use natural low GI sweeteners in moderation. Interestingly, cacao itself is actually good for the teeth because of its high magnesium content and theobromine, which kills the organisms that cause cavities.

MELTING CACAO

Having gone to so much effort to source raw cacao, you need to make sure you melt it gently. You could use a double boiler, but I prefer to not even turn the stove top on. I heat the kettle and place the hot water in a bowl. Then I suspend another bowl with the cacao paste or butter on top of the hot water and wait for it to melt, stirring gently.

If you have an Excalibur dehydrator, you can place your cacao paste and/or butter in a bowl and melt it inside the dehydrator.

WARNINGS

Some people find cacao very stimulating, so adjust consumption according to your experience. Initially, upon discovering that chocolate in its raw state is a health food, over-indulgence is a possibility. Indications of excessive cacao intake include spaciness, ungroundedness, or "rushy" feelings. To balance these effects, drink or eat more greens.

Chocolate is toxic for dogs as they lack the enzymes necessary to metabolize quantities of theobromine in excess of 100–150 mg per kilogram of body weight.

Allergy to chocolate is quite rare. It is more often the case that the person is in fact allergic to milk and dairy products. It is likely that the sugar added to chocolate exacerbates acne.

Because of the large quantity of blood-thinning antioxidants and theobromine in cacao, those on blood-thinning medication need to monitor their bloodwork when introducing cacao into their diets.

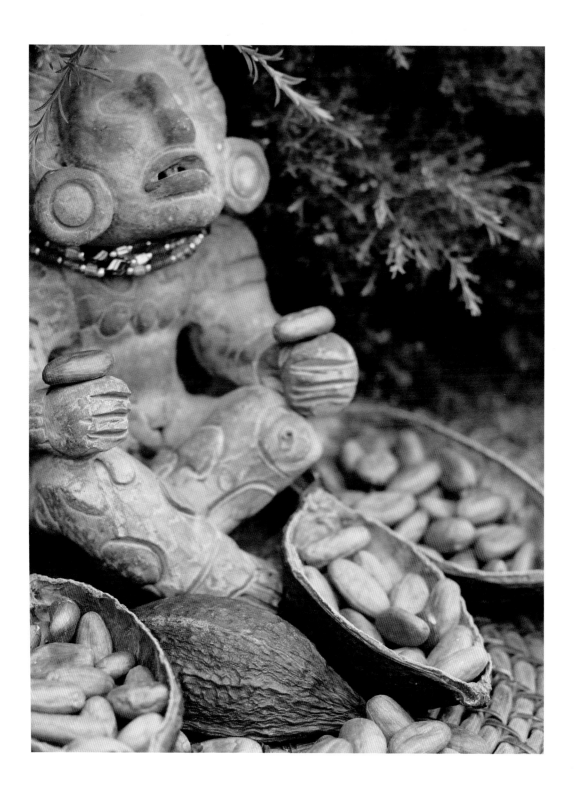

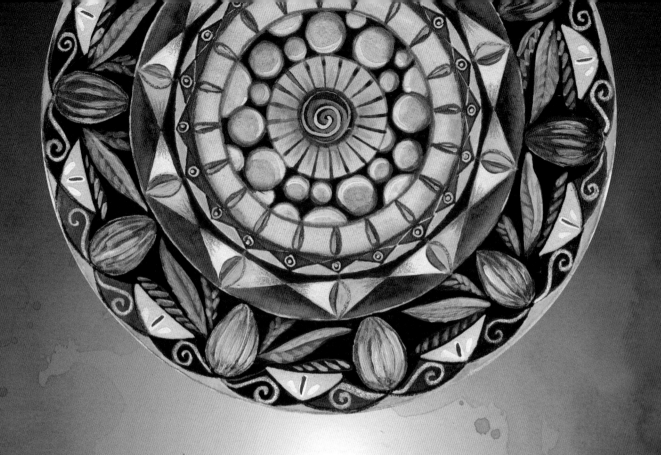

RAW CACAO RECIPES

———————◆———————

CHIA CHOCOLATE BERRY MOUSSE • CHOCOLATE MILK

SIMPLE CHOCOLATE SMOOTHIE • "EVERYTHING'S-IN-IT" SMOOTHIE

CHOCOLATE SAUCE • DECADENT THICK CHOCOLATE SAUCE • HOT CHOCOLATE

CHOCOLATE GANACHE TART WITH SUPERFOOD CRUST

BARBARA'S HAZELNUT FUDGE • CHOCOLATES

———————◆———————

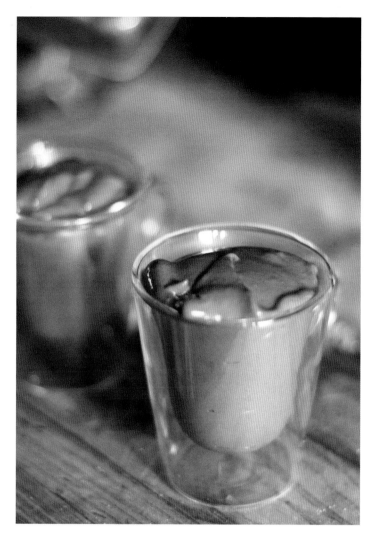

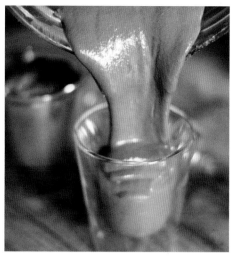

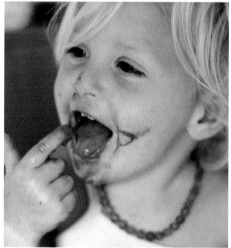

CHIA CHOCOLATE BERRY MOUSSE

Many of our readers will already be familiar with our Rawlicious avocado chocolate mousse, which is simply heavenly. Since discovering chia, we have added this chia chocolate berry mousse to our repertoire of delicious chocolate mousse recipes. This time it's the chia that gives the mousse its thick and creamy texture.

Grind the chia seeds into a fine powder. In a power blender, blend all the ingredients together, and whizz until nice and smooth. Add extra honey for sweetness if desired. Set in the fridge.

Serves 4

½ C chia seeds
2 C water
1 C raw cacao powder
¾ C berries, such as raspberries or strawberries
½ C cashews, soaked
¼ C cacao butter, melted
¼ C of honey
½ T vanilla extract

CHOCOLATE MILK

Makes 2 C

> *2 C hemp milk (see page 131)*
> *3 T cacao powder*
> *honey to taste (optional)*

This is a very simple chocolate milk recipe combining the goodness of cacao and hemp seeds. You can add a banana if you want to turn your chocolate milk into a thicker chocolate shake. You can also see choc omega super-milk (on page 64).

Blend up a batch of hemp milk and add cacao powder. Add honey if extra sweetness is desired.

SIMPLE CHOCOLATE SMOOTHIE

Makes 3 C

> *2 C water*
> *¼ C cashews or Brazil nuts*
> *7 dates*
> *2 T cacao powder*
> *2 T chia seeds*
> *2 T honey*
> *1 T cacao butter*
> *1 T hemp seeds*
> *½ t vanilla powder*
> *pinch of salt*

Blend all the ingredients together. Add ice to cool.

'EVERYTHING'S-IN-IT' SMOOTHIE

Makes ½ gallon

> *2 C water*
> *2 C hemp milk (see page 131)*
> *1 large banana (frozen for cold milkshake)*
> *¼ C dried white mulberries*
> *¼ C raw cacao powder*
> *5 dates*
> *5 Brazil nuts*
> *3 T honey*
> *3 T chia seeds*
> *1 T maca powder*
> *1 T lucuma powder*
> *1 T green powder*
> *1 T mesquite*
> *1 t ashwagandha*
> *1 t astragalus*
> *1 t foti*
> *½ t mucuna*
> *½ t ground cinnamon*
> *1 vanilla pod*
> *1 pinch Himalayan rock salt*

Superfood and superherb chocolate smoothie!

This superfood chocolate smoothie is powered up to extraordinary levels with the superherbs, ashwagandha, astragalus, foti, and mucuna!

Blend everything in a blender. Pour into a flask and enjoy throughout the day.

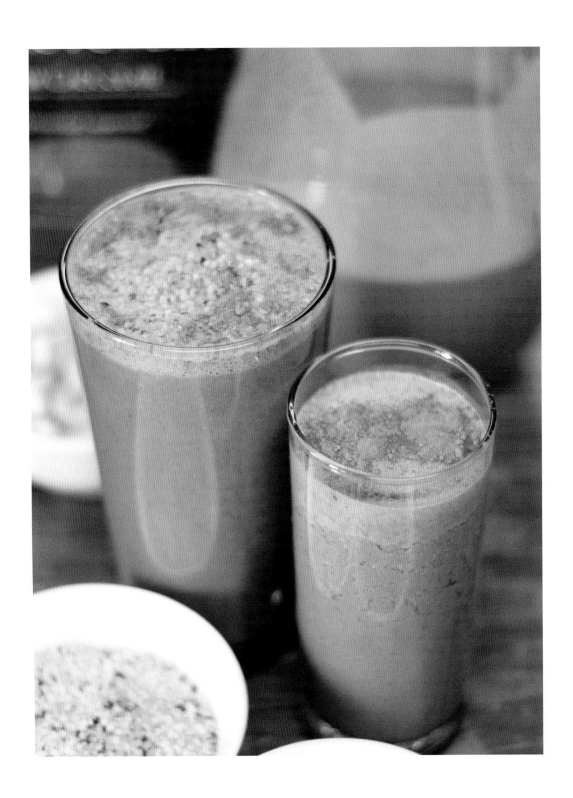

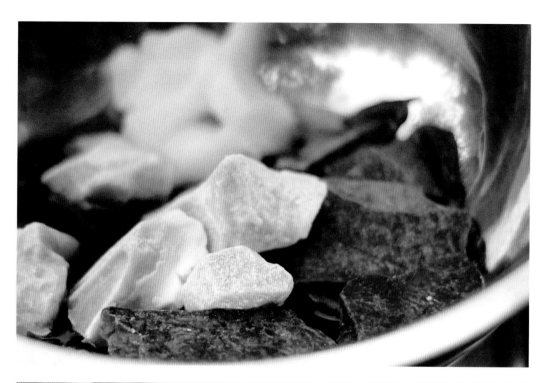

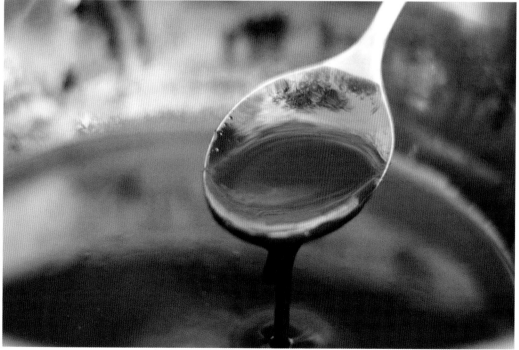

CHOCOLATE SAUCE

This is a simple and quick chocolate sauce recipe.

The cacao paste, butter, and coconut oil in this recipe set immediately on contact with cold foods such as ice cream, making a crisp chocolate "ice cap." This recipe can be made quickly by hand with no blending required.

Makes 1 C

> *½ C cacao paste*
> *¼ C cacao butter*
> *¼ C coconut oil*
> *¼ C maple syrup*

Melt the cacao paste, cacao butter, and coconut oil together and stir in maple syrup.

- -

DECADENT THICK CHOCOLATE SAUCE

This is a more time-consuming recipe than the one above and requires the use of a blender, but it is so worth it! The added nut butter turns it into a decadent, melt-in-your-mouth chocolate experience. It is delicious drizzled over fresh organic strawberries with a chia omega cream (see page 64)!

You can also pour the mixture into a flat dish and turn it into chocolate fudge, adding extra nuts, goji berries, or cacao nibs into the dish for additional texture.

Makes 2 C

> *1 C cacao paste*
> *⅓ C coconut oil*
> *½ C honey*
> *¼ C water*
> *¼ C Brazil nut butter*
> *1–2 T superfoods of choice (optional)*
> *1 t superherbs of choice (optional)*

Melt the cacao paste and coconut oil. Pour into a blender and add the honey and water. Blend on low speed and slowly add the nut butter and any other desired superfoods and superherbs.

HOT CHOCOLATE

The creamy version

Serves 2

> *2 C hot water*
> *¼ C cashews*
> *3 T cacao paste*
> *1 T lucuma powder*
> *2 T honey or coconut sugar*
> *1 T maple syrup*

Blend all ingredients together until smooth.

The ultra-light simple version

Serves 1

> *1¼ C hot water*
> *1 T cacao powder*
> *2 T honey*
> *½ t foti*

Stir all ingredients together in a mug.

The bring-in-more-bliss medicinal version

Serves 2

> *Creamy hot chocolate recipe (above)*

Plus:

> *2 t foti*
> *2 t reishi powder*
> *½ t mucuna*
> *1 t cat's claw*

Make up the creamy hot chocolate recipe above and add the medicinal herbs listed here for a synergistic, mood-enhancing, brain-enlightening experience.

CHOCOLATE GANACHE TART WITH SUPERFOOD CRUST

Serves 10–12

For the superfood crust:

> 2 C pecans
> ¼ C mesquite
> ¼ C lucuma powder
> ¼ C honey
> 3 T coconut oil
> 2 T maca

For the chocolate ganache filling:

> 2 C cashews, soaked for at least
>   30 minutes in warm water,
>   but it's best to soak them
>   overnight
> ½ C maple syrup
> ½ C coconut oil
> ½ C cacao powder
> ¾ C (125 g) cacao paste
> ¾ C water
> 2 t vanilla extract
> a pinch of salt

This is "life by chocolate." The superfood crust is delicious on its own; filled with the chocolate ganache filling, it is out of this world!

In a food processor, pulse all the superfood crust ingredients together to form a crumbly mixture. Press into a quiche tin with a removable base. Prick the base a few times with a fork and place in the fridge while you make up the filling.

In a power blender, blend all the ganache filling ingredients together and pour into the base. Place in the fridge to set for 1 hour.

Serve and *enjoy*!

BARBARA'S HAZELNUT FUDGE

Makes 25 squares

> 1 C hazelnuts
> ½ C cacao paste, melted
> ¼ C cacao butter, melted
> 1 T coconut oil, melted
> ¾ C honey, melted (start with
>   ½ C and add more, up to
>   a ¾ C if you prefer extra
>   sweetness)
> ⅓–½ C nut butter (preferable)
>   or tahini
> ¼ C cacao powder
> 1 t vanilla powder
> a pinch of salt
> extra hazelnuts

This is a hazelnut praline fudge. When our friend Barbara first brought this fudge over for us to try, I thought I was in heaven, so I've asked her to please contribute this recipe to the book.

Put the hazelnuts through the Oscar juicer with the flat plate twice. It will form a crumbed hazelnut paste.

Slowly blend all the melted ingredients together. Add the hazelnut paste, honey, nut butter, cacao powder, vanilla powder, and salt. Blend slowly for a short time. Line a dish with baking paper and pour in the mixture. Sprinkle in extra hazelnuts. Allow to set for 4–6 hours.

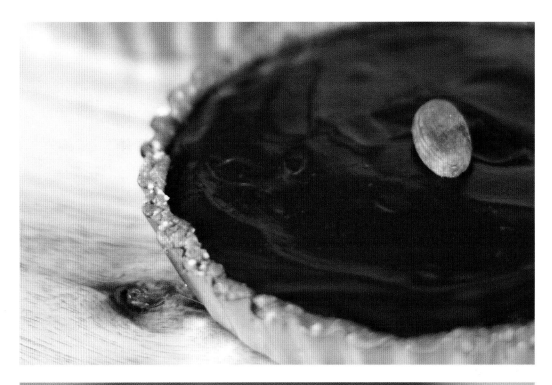

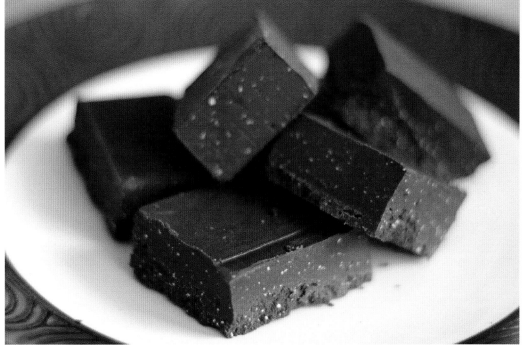

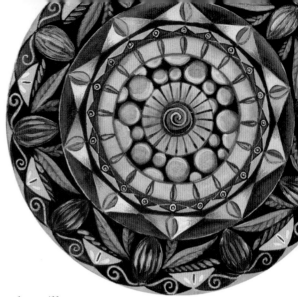

CHOCOLATES

It is easy and fun to make your own raw chocolates. This base chocolate recipe is intended as a platform for your own chocolate creativity. You can play with so many flavor variations; the options are endless.

Commercial chocolate uses trans fats, dairy, and sugar, but when you make chocolate using superfoods such as raw cacao, honey, or maple syrup and coconut oil, you are creating superfood nutrition with the world's favorite food—chocolate, the food of the gods!

> ⅞ C (200 g) cacao paste
> ½ C (100 g) cacao butter
> ¼ C coconut oil
> ¼ C honey
> flavoring and/or superfoods (optional)

Melt the cacao paste, cacao butter, and coconut oil and put in your power blender. Add the honey and blend on low speed. All the ingredients can be mixed through by hand if you do not have a power blender.

Add the flavoring and/or superfoods of your choice and pour into chocolate molds or ice trays and allow to set in the fridge. Here are some of my favorite flavor combinations:

Rose geranium and goji

Add 1 drop of rose geranium essential oil and a handful of gojis.

Mint and spirulina

Add 1 drop of mint essential oil and 1 t spirulina powder, and all you will taste is the mint—not a hint of spirulina!

Maca and vanilla

Add 1 T maca and 1 t vanilla extract.

Lucuma and orange

Add 1 T lucuma powder and 1 drop of orange essential oil.

Other options

You could also add:
mesquite
ginger essential oil
cardamom

Medicinal herbs

Cacao is traditionally used as a carrier of medicine. Add any or all of the following medicinal herbs to the base chocolate mixture for your very own medicinal chocolates:

> 1 t reishi powder
> ½ t ashwagandha
> 1 t astragalus
> ⅛ t sceletium
> ¼ t red ginseng
> ½ t taheebo
> ¼ t cat's claw
> ½ t Siberian ginseng
> 1 T foti
> ½ t cayenne pepper
> a pinch of salt

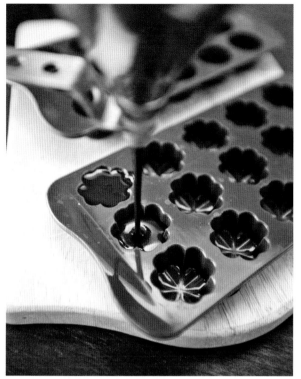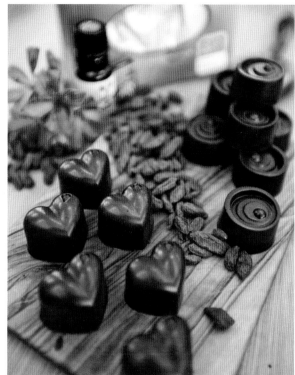
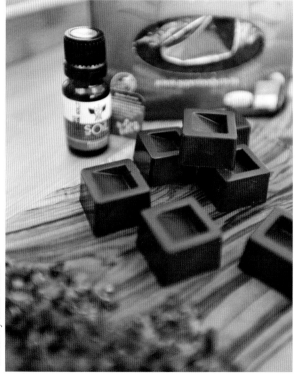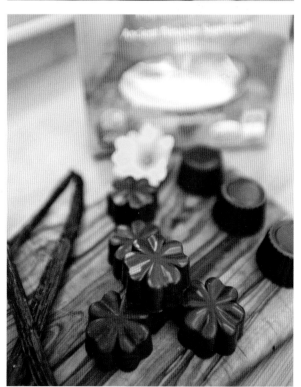

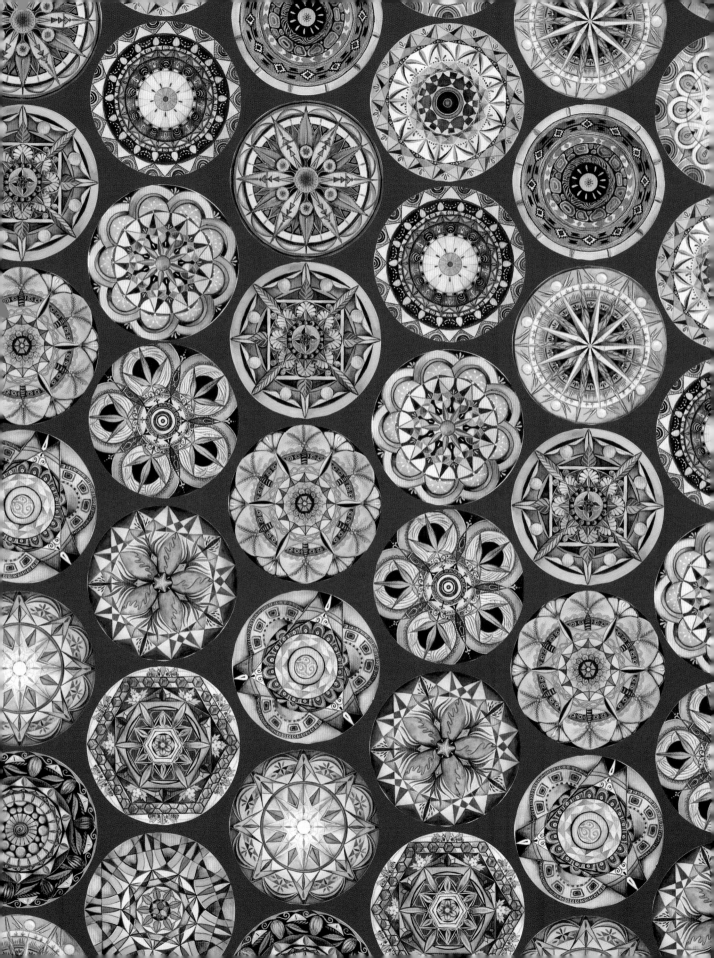

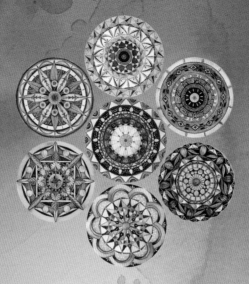

MEDICINAL HERBS

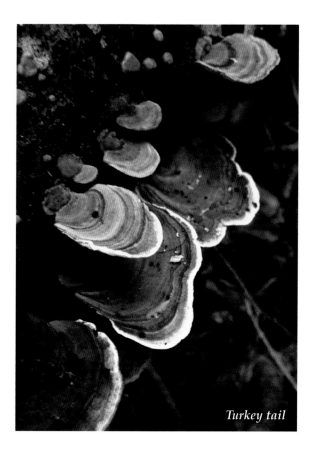

Turkey tail

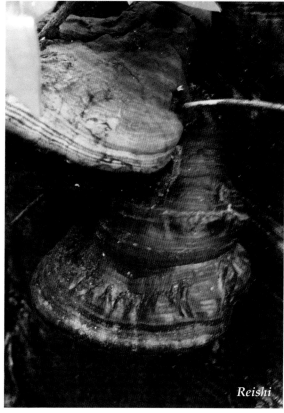

Reishi

MEDICINAL HERBS

Superherbs are herbs that traditional healing systems such as Chinese medicine, Ayurveda, African herbalism, and Amazonian herbalism have incorporated for thousands of years for their powerful healing effects. Most people are well below a functional baseline of health and well on their way to disease, or already challenged by many disease symptoms. Medicinal herbs are essential in these situations, but they also act as preventatives for those who are already following a healthy lifestyle.

Traditionally used medicinal herbs known to be adaptogens can restore the body to balance better than any medicine, because they target and strengthen the whole body. The Chinese definition of a tonic herb is anything that you can consume on a daily basis over the long term without negative side effects (while being kept within a reasonable dosage). Tonic herbal adaptogens are non-specific because they balance and tone (quite different from boosting or suppressing) a wide range of different biological functions all at once.

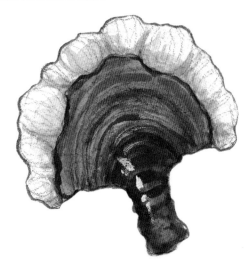

HOW WE USE TONIC HERBS

Tonic herbs are usually sold as powder to make tea from, but can also be found as capsules or tinctures. We like to add the powders to our superfood smoothies, and we regularly have a pot of tonic herb tea going with mushrooms that we wild-harvested ourselves. These are potent medicinal herbs, so we suggest starting with a small dose, as little as a quarter of a teaspoon. Once familiar with their effect, dosage can be increased to 1–2 teaspoons.

What follows is a list of some of the most common, well-studied, and widely used medicinal herbs.

MEDICINAL MUSHROOMS

Reishi

Reishi has been the most revered herbal mushroom in Asia for over two thousand years. The Taoists consider it an "elixir of immortality" that increases the spiritual *shen* energy. Reishi has been proven effective in aiding the treatment of arthritis, and it possesses anti-allergenic, anti-inflammatory, antiviral, antibacterial, and antioxidant properties. Reishi is also an excellent anti-stress herb, known to ease tension, elevate the spirit, and promote peace of mind by transforming negative energy in the body.

Chaga

Chaga is a highly prized tonic mushroom, long used in traditional Siberian, Korean, Chinese, Northern European, and Scandinavian herbalism. It is found growing wild in old forests throughout the colder regions of Northern Asia and Northern Europe. Asian herbalists believe that Siberian chaga preserves youthfulness and promotes health and longevity. Chaga is the King of the Medicinal Mushrooms. It contains the highest amounts of anti-tumor, cancer-fighting compounds of any herb.

Chaga is also extremely high in nourishing phytochemicals, nutrients, and free radical–scavenging antioxidants.

Maitake

Maitake is prized in traditional Chinese and Japanese herbalism as a medicinal mushroom, used to balance out stressed body systems to normal levels. Maitake contains polysaccharides that stimulate the immune system and has the ability to regulate blood pressure, glucose, insulin, and both serum and liver lipids such as cholesterol, triglycerides, and phospholipids, and may also be useful for weight loss. Research also suggests powerful anti-tumor properties.

Turkey tail

Turkey tail mushrooms are one of the most researched and respected of the medicinal mushrooms. They are also one of the most common in the northern forests of the world, from Europe to China and Japan, from Siberia to the United States and Canada. Turkey tail mushrooms are medically significant for many reasons. They are anti-microbial, immunomodulating, antioxidant, and anti-malarial, but they are most popularly known as being the natural source of the anticarcinogenic polysaccharide (PSK). PSK is a high molecular weight carbohydrate found in the fruitbodies and in the mycelium of turkey tail mushrooms.

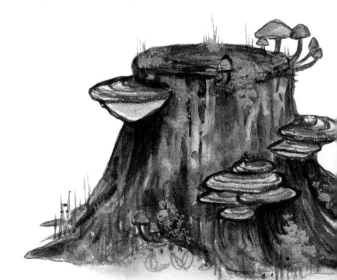

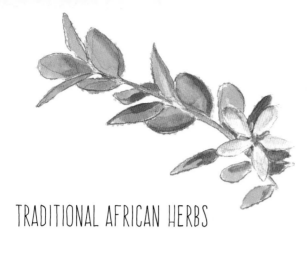

TRADITIONAL AFRICAN HERBS

Although not strictly tonic herbs, these African medicinal herbs can be safely used if and when needed. Most are sold with directions for use.

Buchu

Buchu is one of South Africa's best-known medicinal plants and has been used by the indigenous peoples of the area for centuries to treat a wide range of ailments. The leaves of the buchu plant are an effective diuretic and are antimicrobial and anti-inflammatory. These medicinal properties make buchu effective in the treatment of bladder infections, urinary tract infections, and kidney infections. Buchu is also often used to treat prostate infections.

Devil's claw

Devil's claw originates from the Kalahari Desert and savannah regions of south and southeast Africa. In these parts of the world, devil's claw has historically been used to treat a wide range of conditions, including fever, malaria, and indigestion. This herb has an extensive history of use as an anti-inflammatory, pain reliever, and digestive stimulant. Devil's claw offers slow but sure relief of joint pain caused by osteoarthritis or rheumatoid arthritis, and has also been shown to relieve muscle pain and enhance mobility for people with either arthritis or muscle injuries.

Sceletium

Sceletium tortuosum is a rare succulent found in certain semi-desert areas of southern Africa. It is highly regarded and sought after by both the Khoikhoi and the San people, who have used this plant as a mood enhancer since prehistoric times. Sceletium elevates mood and decreases anxiety, stress, and tension, and is a very effective antidepressant. Sceletium is known to reduce addictive cravings, particularly with regard to nicotine, and also lessens the withdrawal effects of alcohol and other addictive drugs. It also helps balance aberrant brain chemistry caused by the effects of serotonin-depleting drugs.

Sutherlandia

Sutherlandia frutescens is regarded as one of the most profound and multi-purpose of the medicinal plants in southern Africa. It has enjoyed a long history of use as a safe and efficacious remedy for diverse health conditions by all cultures in the region. It has long been used as a supportive treatment in cancer, hence one of its common names: cancer bush or *kankerbos*.

African ginger

The highly aromatic roots of this rare southern African plant are regarded as Africa's foremost natural anti-inflammatory remedy. It has a long history of use in African traditional medicine for a range of conditions, including headaches, colds and flu, mild asthma, sinusitis, throat infections, and bad breath. It is considered an excellent antiseptic, circulatory stimulant, and overall body detoxifier. It is a mild sedative, balancing mood swings and calming hysteria. It has an expectorant effect on the lungs, expelling phlegm and relieving coughs and chest infections. It relieves colic, abdominal pain, and spasm, and helps to relieve griping caused by diarrhea. It is good for PMS, relaxes menstrual cramping, promotes menstruation, and helps with delayed and scanty periods. It also relieves painful ovulation and is used to invigorate the reproductive system generally.

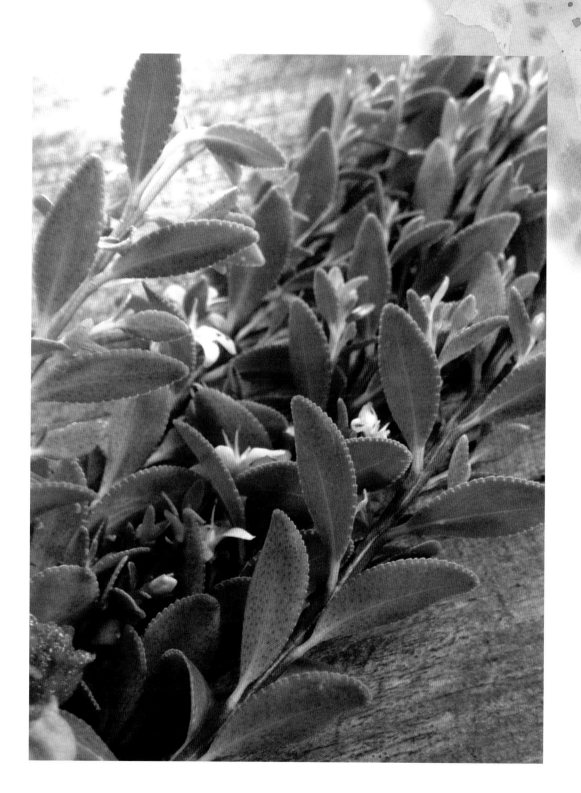

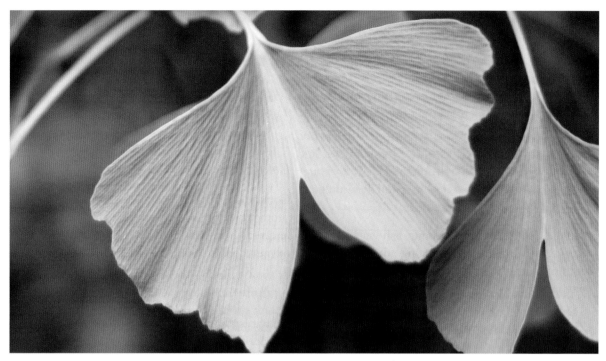

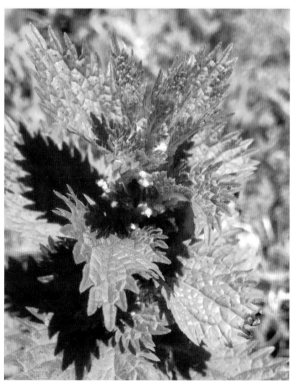

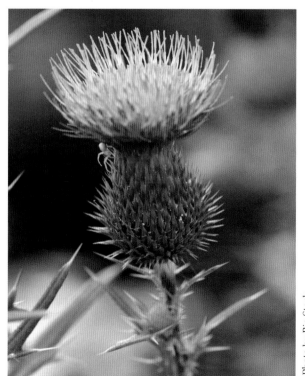

TRADITIONAL SOUTH AMERICAN HERBS

Pau d'arco or taheebo

Pau d'arco is an herb found in the rainforests of the Amazon and other parts of South America. Pau d'arco bark has been used by indigenous peoples for centuries to address a spectrum of health problems. Pau d'arco is commonly used to support indications of allergies, liver problems, and candida and yeast infections. It has powerful antifungal, antibacterial, and antiviral properties, which makes it a perfect herb for cleaning parasites and candida out of the body.

Cat's claw

Cat's claw grows as a vine in the Amazon, where the root bark is stripped off and made into herbal teas. Also known as "uña de gato," cat's claw is probably the most revered medicinal herb in all of South American herbalism. Cat's claw is renowned for its anti-inflammatory and analgesic properties. It has been used for many years in the treatment of inflammatory processes associated with arthritis and rheumatism and also in the treatment of gastrointestinal disorders such as gastritis and gastric ulcers. It boosts the immune system and helps in the treatment of viral and other microbial infections. Cat's claw is a powerful antioxidant and is thought to be useful in the treatment of some cancers.

Chanca piedra

This South American herb has traditionally been used to eliminate gallbladder and kidney stones. The English translation for "chanca piedra" is "stone crusher."

TRADITIONAL NORTH AMERICAN HERBS

Milk thistle

Milk thistle has been used medicinally for over two thousand years, most commonly for the treatment of liver and gallbladder disorders.

Slippery elm bark

Slippery elm is a tree native to North America. It is the inner bark that has medicinal value. It is a demulcent, emollient, expectorant, and diuretic. Demulcent means that it is soothing, softening, buffering, and has poison-drawing qualities. It helps to neutralize stomach acids, boost the adrenal glands, and draw out impurities.

Nettle root and leaf

The nettle leaf and root both have medicinal properties but are more effective against different complaints respectively. Nettle root is used as a treatment for prostate problems, which often affect men from about the age of forty. Nettle leaves are also thought to have many beneficial anti-inflammatory properties. They help reduce inflammation in the urinary tract. They act as a diuretic, helping to cleanse and improve bladder and kidney functions. Nettles have also been used to help combat common allergies such as hay fever. Studies have shown that nettles have antihistamine properties, which may help reduce allergy symptoms such as sneezing and itching. Nettles may also help reduce certain skin inflammations such as eczema.

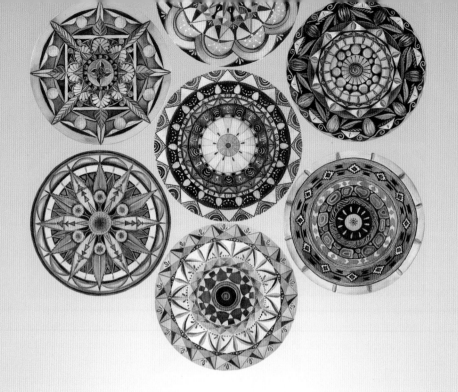

RESOURCES

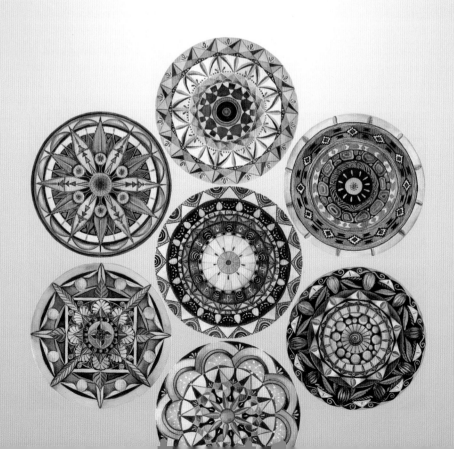

RAWLICIOUS: RECIPES FOR RADIANT HEALTH

by Peter and Beryn Daniel

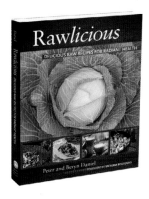

Rawlicious is our first raw food recipe book, first published in South Africa in 2009 and in the United States in 2011. As raw food chefs, our primary motivation is the long-term health benefits of the food we make and eat. At the same time, we realize that enjoying food is an important and natural part of the experience. When food tastes delicious, it is easy to eat! What you will find inside *Rawlicious* is a collection of simple, new, and interesting ways to prepare and enjoy raw plant foods.

RAWLICIOUS

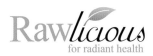

Join the Rawlicious family.
Sign up for our newsletter at www.rawlicious.co.za to hear more about:
- free talks
- other Rawlicious events
- new and exciting superfoods we have found
- fantastic seasonal raw food and superfood discounts
- special offers on equipment

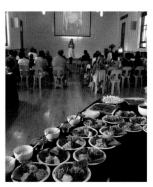

Rawlicious events

We have been educating people about the benefits of raw foods and superfoods via our Rawlicious events for over seven years now. We regularly run free lecture evenings and Rawlicious seminars.

You can find a current schedule of events at www.rawlicious.co.za.

RAWLICIOUS DVD COURSE

Now you can take our Rawlicious course from the comfort of your own home and kitchen! The Rawlicious DVD course is a complete introduction to the Rawlicious raw food lifestyle. It covers a broad spectrum of recipes and raw principles, from basics such as sprouting, juicing, detoxification, and cleansing to salad preparation, soups, and smoothies, as well as more advanced gourmet recipes. There are also healthy raw desserts and chocolates for some healthy, indulgent fun.

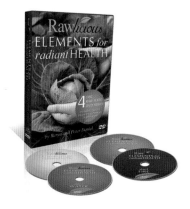

Special interviews with people who have experienced increased energy, improved peak performance, extreme weight loss, and greater health and happiness are guaranteed to inspire.

For more information, visit www.rawlicious.co.za.

WEBSHOP

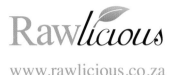

www.rawlicious.co.za

We have a user-friendly, secure webshop that sells directly to the public at www.rawlicious.co.za. Over and above our own Superfoods brand, we have sourced other superfoods, super-supplements, and raw food items from local suppliers that support ongoing health. We only stock products that we are happy to use ourselves. Every ingredient that we refer to in this book is either readily or seasonally available at your local grocer, health food store, our Superfoods shop, or via our webshop. If you can't find something, we will most likely be able to source it for you.

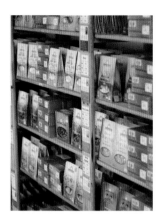

VISIT OUR SUPERFOODS SHOP AND RAWLICIOUS DELI

Our Soaring Free Superfoods headquarters and shop are located in Cape Town. Our Superfoods shop and Rawlicious deli stock a full range of superfoods, wholefood supplements, kitchen equipment, and accessories, as well as raw food smoothies, chocolates, snacks, and treats. Please feel free to pop in, browse, shop, connect, and chat.

Our shop team is available to demonstrate how to use the healthy lifestyle equipment, such as power blenders, juicers, or dehydrators, at any time during shop hours.

Call 0861 000 976 or visit our website for directions. For calls outside South Africa, dial +27 21 702 4980.

FACEBOOK AND TWITTER

Visit and like our Facebook page (Rawlicious) or follow us on Twitter (@RawliciousTribe). Our Facebook page is a hub of activity that will help you keep your finger on the pulse of what is happening in this new and exciting realm of cutting-edge nutrition.

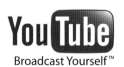

YOUTUBE

Check out our YouTube channel (RawliciousTribe). Peter regularly uploads videos of our free talks, as well as informational videos about superfoods and so much more!

THE SUPERFOODS BRAND

www.superfoods.co.za

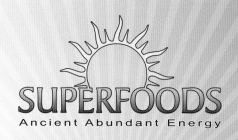

When we returned to South Africa, we found that many of the superfoods that we were accustomed to eating while we lived abroad were not available. We started importing our favorite superfoods—goji berries and cacao were the first—mainly to keep ourselves and our friends in good supply. Very soon, we were supplying the people in our workshops, then local health shops, specialized delis, and so on. We created our own brand dedicated to sourcing and distributing only the highest-quality organic superfoods we could find. We now have a wide and continuously growing range of superfoods available both in retail and bulk options.

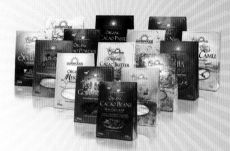

We pride ourselves on being purveyors of the finest-tasting and most health-enhancing certified organic superfoods in the world! Not only does our raw cacao, for example, come from the best organic raw cacao beans, they are also cold-processed—something quite rare in the industry. This preserves their rawness and the sensitive cacao nutrients and phytonutrients inherent within the raw bean. Superfoods such as heirloom cacao also preserve forests as they grow better when planted under the forest canopy. Supporting a certified organic brand also supports indigenous farmers who grow certified organic food.

We love living a superfood raw lifestyle and are always looking for new ways to make it even simpler for others to enjoy it with us. Many people tell us they wish they could eat like we do. All too often we hear things such as: "I'd love to, but it's too difficult to make," or "It's too time-consuming," or "It's so expensive," or "Won't you come and live in my house and do it for me?" People really do want to eat healthier, but with busy days, work, and family commitments, it comes down to: "If only you would prepare the food for us." So that's what we've done!

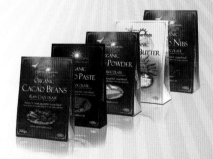

CHIA MEAL FOR BREAKFAST
TRAIL MIX FOR SNACKING
GREEN SHAKE FOR ALKALIZING
SUPERSHAKE FOR ENERGY

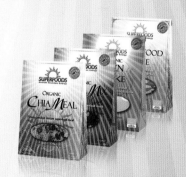

Ramp up your superfood consumption with these superfood mixes and enjoy the magical unfolding journey toward radiant health along with us.

EQUIPMENT

When it comes to a juicer, blender, dehydrator, or food processor, there are many to choose from across a broad price range.

Choosing the best and the most practical

There's nothing worse than buying an expensive piece of kitchen equipment, only to realize that if you'd spent just a little bit extra you would have had a better and more practical machine.

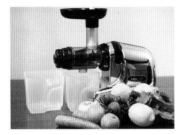

Juicer

The Oscar: This is a single-gear masticating juicer, meaning that it grinds up your fruit or vegetable slowly against a juicing screen instead of spinning it like a centrifugal juicer would. This means that you get more of the goodness out of the produce. It juices all fruits and vegetables, including green leafy vegetables and wheatgrass. It comes with a handy crushing screen, and it's quiet and easy to clean.

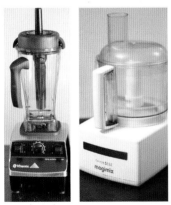
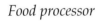

Blender

The Vitamix: This is a high-speed power blender that will change your life. You can put wet and dry ingredients into the jug and blend, grind, powder, pulverize, chop, mince, puree, or crush various ingredients.

Food processor

The Magimix: This food processor is the top-of-the-range, sturdy, all-purpose chopping and mixing appliance. It comes with useful grating and slicing attachments.

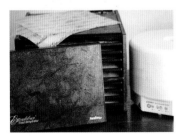

Dehydrator

The Excalibur or Ezi-dri: A dehydrator is a glorified hairdryer. It has a fan at the bottom that blows and circulates warm air through the trays. The two brands mentioned here are dehydrators that allow you to set the drying temperature to your desired setting. Remember: It is important to warm or dry your food at low temperatures so as not to destroy the enzymes, nutrients, and vitamins. There is no point in buying a cheap dehydrator that only has one drying setting of over 158°F (70°C).

All of the above-mentioned equipment comes with reliable guarantees, servicing options, and replaceable parts.

Visit our Superfoods shop for a demonstration, call us on 0861 000 976 or visit www.rawlicious.co.za for more information or to place an order. For calls outside South Africa, dial +27 21 702 4980.

RECOMMENDED READING

There are many inspirational books on superfoods and raw foods to continue exploring. Here are some of the ones you will find on our bookshelf:

Rawlicious: Recipes for Radiant Health by Peter and Beryn Daniel

The Sunfood Diet Success System by David Wolfe

Superfoods by David Wolfe

Naked Chocolate by David Wolfe

Chaga: King of the Medicinal Mushrooms by David Wolfe

Longevity Now: A Comprehensive Approach to Healthy Hormones, Detoxification, Super Immunity, Reversing Calcification, and Total Rejuvenation by David Wolfe

Easy Living Food by Natalie Reid and Noel Marten

Recipes from Our Organic Garden by Antonia DeLuca

Conscious Eating by Gabriel Cousens

The Ancient Wisdom of the Chinese Tonic Herbs by Ron Teeguarden

Wheatgrass — Nature's Finest Medicine by Steve Meyerowitz

Green for Life by Victoria Boutenko

Chia: Rediscovering a Forgotten Crop of the Aztecs by Ricardo Ayerza and Wayne Coates

Goji: The Himalayan Health Secret by Dr. Earl Mindell

Wolfberry: Nature's Bounty of Nutrition and Health by P.M. Gross

The Coconut Oil Miracle by Bruce Fife

Hemp for Health: The Medicinal and Nutritional Uses of Cannabis Sativa by Chris Conrad

The Great Book of Hemp: The Complete Guide to the Environmental, Commercial, and Medicinal Uses of the World's Most Extraordinary Plant by Rowan Robinson

The Sprouting Book: How to Grow and Use Sprouts to Maximize Your Health and Vitality by Ann Wigmore

Fats That Heal, Fats That Kill by Udo Erasmus

THE RAW FOOD AND SUPERFOOD MOVEMENT

There is a fast-growing worldwide community of raw food–eating, health-conscious people. A change of lifestyle such as the one described in this book can seem extreme and isolating at first, but when we scratch the surface just a little bit, we find rich and fertile soil: like-minded people who are embracing change, willing to connect, and wanting to create supportive and sustainable communities that touch and tread lightly on the earth.

Reach out and connect.

To your health, joy, and freedom.

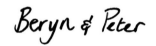

CONTACT DETAILS

www.rawlicious.co.za
www.superfoods.co.za

Superfoods

Office hours: 9 a.m.–4 p.m.
Tel: 0861 000976
International tel: +27 21 702 4980
Fax: +27 21 702 4970
Email: info@rawlicious.co.za

Postal address

PostNet Suite 354, Private bag X16, Constantia, 7848, Cape Town, South Africa

INDEX

C

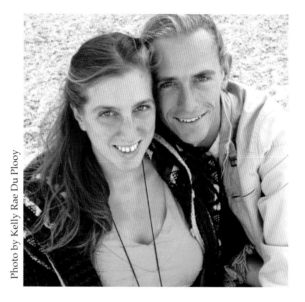

Photo by Kelly Rae Du Plooy

ABOUT THE AUTHORS

Peter and Beryn Daniel are founders of the raw food and superfood movements in South Africa, raw food chefs, authors of *Rawlicious: Delicious Recipes for Radiant Health,* and producers of the four-part *Rawlicious, Elements for Radiant Health* DVD course.

Initially introduced to superfoods and raw foods while living in the UK, Peter and Beryn first came across goji berries, and a short while later, in search of an alternative to mass-marketed chocolate, they discovered raw cacao online. These superfoods changed their lives. As soon as they realized that eating healthily included delicious and indulgent taste sensations, they embarked on their raw food and superfoods journey with vigor.

Since then, their superfoods journey has led them to many remote and exciting places: from the cacao jungles of Ecuador, to Peru, to the deep Gobi Desert, behind the Himalayas in China in search of wild gojis, and the wild African bush for *aloe ferox* and ancient baobabs. Superfoods such as maca, chia seeds, wheatgrass, hemp, and many other superherbs and medicinal mushrooms have found their way into their lives and their alchemical kitchen.

Peter and Beryn have been presenting workshops and seminars on the rawlicious superfood lifestyle for over seven years and have been ingesting the nutritional potency of superfoods for even longer. They live in Cape Town with their daughter Katara.